Calories & Corsets

Calories & Corsets

A history of dieting over 2,000 years

Louise Foxcroft

P

PROFILE BOOKS

First published in Great Britain in 2011 by
PROFILE BOOKS LTD
3A Exmouth House
Pine Street
London ECIR OJH
www.profilebooks.com

1 3 5 7 9 10 8 6 4 2

Typeset in Garamond by MacGuru Ltd
info@macguru.org.uk
Printed and bound in Great Britain by
Clays, Bungay, Suffolk

A CIP catalogue record for this book is available from the British Library.

ISBN 978 1 84668 425 8
eISBN 978 1 84765 458 8

The paper this book is printed on is certified by the © 1996 Forest
Stewardship Council A.C. (FSC). It is ancient-forest friendly. The printer
holds FSC chain of custody SGS-COC-2061

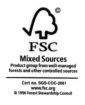

FSC
Mixed Sources
Product group from well-managed
forests and other controlled sources
Cert no. SGS-COC-2061
www.fsc.org
© 1996 Forest Stewardship Council

Virtually all so-called obesity cures … are simply shrewd schemes for fooling the overweight, and the purchasers of most of them are being kidded by experts.

Arthur J. Cramp, 'Fooling the Fat' in
Your Weight and How to Control it (1928)

I have always wanted a mistress who was fat.

Paul Gauguin (1848–1903)

If fat is not an insidious creeping enemy, I do not know what is.

William Banting, *Letter on Corpulence,
Addressed to the Public* (1869)

To the scientist there is nothing so tragic on earth as the sight of a fat man eating a potato.

Vance Thompson, 1920s

Whatever be the quantity that a man eats, it is plain that if he is too fat, he has eaten more than he should have done.

Samuel Johnson (1709–84)

That fat men are indolent and stupid is well recognised.

Leonard Williams, MD, *Obesity* (1926)

A fat man is a joke, and a fat woman is two jokes – one on herself and one on her husband.

Cecil Webb-Johnson, MD, *Why Be Fat?* (1923)

Are you aware that fatness has destroyed your sex appeal and made you look older, somewhat like a buffoon whom people are inclined not to take seriously in any area or on any level?

Frank J. Wilson, *Glamour, Glucose and Glands* (1956)

For my dad and his love of words

CONTENTS

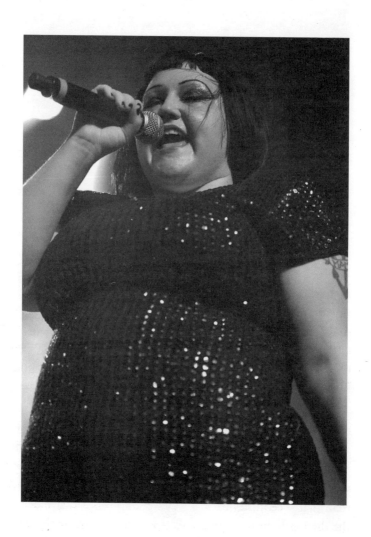

1. Too many of us are labouring under the tyranny of a culturally prescribed body shape; where dieting is the norm and a skinny body the goal. Women such as the singer Beth Ditto are facing down the prejudice and the bullying and challenging today's ideas of what is beautiful. She has used her weight to promote her belief that 'such a personal thing as one's body should never be a reason for controversy, since every person is beautiful in their own way'. The story of beauty and the story of health have always been intertwined but the long and mean history of body-shaping and diets has distorted our view of both.

1

Introduction: 'The Price of a Boyish Form'

F AT, PLUMP, STOUT, overweight, large, chubby, portly, flabby, paunchy, pot-bellied, beer-bellied, meaty, of ample proportions, heavyset, obese, corpulent, fleshy, gross, plus-sized, big-boned, tubby, roly-poly, well-upholstered, beefy, porky, blubbery, chunky, pudgy, podgy, bulky, substantial, voluminous, voluptuous, generous, lardy … We've heard them all.

Fat is 'bad' and dieting is the new norm, but few people in recent decades have had what we might call a 'normal' relationship with food, one untouched by the constant barrage of diet news, fast foods and a food environment radically different from what it was even just a generation ago. If we look further back than that – centuries back – it becomes obvious that much of the dieting industry is fraudulent, yet still we follow the latest fad, hoping for some quick and easy weight-loss miracle because slimming down is hard, tedious work. Our attitudes to our bodies, and to fat and food, need to change.

Fad diets are little better than useless. They do the biggest business and arguably the greatest harm, and they have been around since long before your great-grandmother was eyeing up that fetching knitted knee-length number for her trip to Bognor with a new beau. Dieters can initially lose 5 to 10 per cent of their weight on any number of fad diets, but the weight almost always comes back. A recent report by the American Psychological Association which looked at thirty-one diet studies found that, after two years of dieting, up to two-thirds of dieters weighed more than they did before they began their regimen. Sustained weight loss was found only in a small minority of the participants, while complete weight regain was found in the majority. Diets, they concluded, 'do not lead to sustained weight loss or health benefits for the majority of people'. And there is evidence that yo-yo dieting is something of a Faustian bargain: it can make the whole enterprise more difficult so that repeat dieters find they have to eat less and for longer to lose the same amount of weight. Recent evidence suggests that, even though the most important changes we can make to reduce our cancer risk (after giving up smoking) are to exercise and lose weight, repeated dieting is linked to cardiovascular disease, stroke, diabetes and a compromised immune system. The human cost of both obesity and yo-yo crash dieting is bad enough but there are huge economic costs too. We need to re-think our quest for unrealistic thinness through sometimes dangerous, expensive and misguided crash diets and pills, and return to a simple, sensible healthy approach to eating as first set out by the Greeks.

While I was writing this, and feeling a bit of a fraud because I've never seriously attempted a diet, I had a go at a low-carbohydrate plan to see how it would feel and whether I'd be able to stick it out. It was a strict regimen that I got from a best-selling diet book, and it proved to be much more of a trial than I'd imagined. I'm not by nature an obsessive person but from the minute I woke up each day I found myself thinking about food. I thought about what I could eat, when I could eat it, how much I could have and, particularly insidious, I cast sideways glances at friends and family to check on what everyone else was having.

I took to weighing myself – naked, before my first cup of coffee, and then clothed, and then late, after dinner at night, just so I could obtain the greatest range of numbers and ruminate on where I was in my diet and what it all meant (answer: very little, other than I lost half a pound, but all this weighing and obsessing proved a major distraction from the work that I should have been getting on with). What it did provide was a real insight into the way in which dieting can become obsessive and how any new diet that promises stress-free, painless and fast weight loss is instantly attractive. The repetitive and often unsatisfying experience of dieting can only be debunked by a long, hard look at its history, a process that could release us from the tyranny of fads and quick-fixes.

What can a look at centuries of dieting, gluttony, abstinence and artifice tell us about tried and tested (or used and abused) diets and regimens? Such a survey will range from the ideal Greek body to the celebration of plump flesh by medicine and the arts in times of dearth; from the industrialisation of society, which brought new foods, fashions and stigmas, to wartime scarcity and political constraints; from the rounded hour-glass figures of 1950s 'sweater girls' to the insubstantial and boyish Twiggy-type. From heroin chic, Kate Moss in her pants and the size zero debate, to the explosion of magazines and websites such as *Heat* and *TMZ*, the ideal woman has become smaller, skinnier and more sickly as real women have gained their independence and got bigger. Sifting through all the accumulated centuries of advice and instruction, science and psychology, insanity and innovation we will discover the often really wild truth about dieting. All the errors and attitudes, shapes and *Schadenfreude*, sense and nonsense of dieting will be laid bare and might even put to rest the notion that there is a magic dieting 'something' which stands out from all the fads and fashions, and which has THIS WORKS stamped all over it.

*

In 1953, three years before I was born, Simone de Beauvoir wrote, 'One is not born, but rather becomes, a woman.' As I grew up in tandem with feminism I absorbed the idea that feminist theory begins with the body, that everything has been written on the body: all the inequalities, the prejudices, the rights and wrongs. Not only is your body inescapable, but what society says about it is, too, and what we regard as 'nature' is, in fact, socially constructed. Our perception of our bodies changes over time and each period and every culture has had its own obsession with a particular body shape, with appearance, with what is seen as beautiful or ugly. Add to this the fact that as we age our bodies change shape, and the notion of attractiveness becomes evermore nuanced. Desirable body shapes are culturally specific and prejudice is heaped upon those whose bodies differ; and this norm, this marker of beauty and belonging, has continually altered. Modern feminism, operating now in the interests of both women and men, is of course still trying to remove these prejudices, to liberate us all from convention.

When I was ten years old, in 1966, at a family party an uncle remarked on how I was growing and serenaded me with a medley of Maurice Chevalier songs. He began with 'Every little breeze seems to whisper "Louise", Birds in the trees …' and moved on, creepily crooning in his mock Gallic accent, to 'Thank Heaven for little girls (they grow up in the most delightful way)'. Then he asked what I wanted to be when I grew up. Happily occupying his warm worsted lap and enveloped in the powerful, pungent smell of men – of whisky and tobacco and Brylcreem – I cocked my head, swung my pigtails, and answered, 'Miss World.' That seemed to me then to be the epitome of female achievement. I already knew that all the female characters in the British children's television programmes of the time were passive, silent or fixed to the spot: Louby Lou, Little Weed and the Wooden Top mother and daughter. By contrast the Miss World contestants were visible: they spoke (after a fashion), and they were out there getting a lot of attention. They had grown-up 'ideal' female bodies, but they acted and stood like girls: coquettish, showing off but disguising it by holding their heads to one side, apparently ever so malleable, demure in their fitted swimsuits and white high heels. They were catching men. I could already identify with them, with the way that they were obviously one thing pretending to be another; their real selves camouflaged in order to succeed in a skewed world. It was clear, even to a child, that you needed to look the part, and in the early 1960s that part involved big pointy breasts, a nipped-in waist and round hips. Their 'vital statistics' were all-important, with 36, 24, 36 the preferred incantation. So as a young girl I already believed that beauty could be measured and worked for, and the rewards were many. When I grew up I would work on my body so that I, too, could sit on more men's laps and bask.

Then in 1970, when I turned fourteen, the Miss World competition was brought to a chaotic halt by a band of noisy feminists. The presenter that year, Bob Hope, was taken aback by flying tomatoes, flour bombs, ink, and angry shouts of 'cattle market'. Bob's conclusion was that the protesters he faced must have been 'on some kind of dope'. Ha! Watching it all on television, I can't tell you how exciting, indeed how joyously radical it was to see and hear the women chanting, 'We're not beautiful, we're not ugly, we're angry.' That year, too, the Equal Pay Act was passed in Britain, three years after David Steel's Abortion Act. In America in 1971, the National Women's Political Caucus (NWPC) was founded by Gloria Steinem, Betty Friedan and Bella Abzug, and in 1972 the Equal Rights Amendment was passed by the Senate at much the same time that *Ms.* magazine was launched. I no longer saw any need to be sugar and spice, I had a boyfriend, twenty-four to my sixteen, who thought me worryingly 'precocious', and by the time the Sex Discrimination Act was passed in 1975 I was nineteen, in London, on the Pill, with no make-up, no bra, no knickers, no razor, *Spare Rib* under my arm, my sisters by my side – and feminist to the bone.

Yet, as I became a young woman in the midst of feminism's second wave, we were all still labouring under the tyranny of a prescribed body shape. Many of us refused to succumb, but I look back now knowing that it was easy enough to do so then, for we were young and therefore, almost by definition, beautiful. Thirty-odd years ago, in my early twenties, I had two babies. I got BIG. When I gained three stone, only seven pounds or so of which was baby, my doctor gave me a sternly paternal lecture on how much fat I was putting on. He told me, with great confidence, in fact, that I 'would blow up like a barrage balloon' and that I'd struggle to lose the weight if I insisted on breastfeeding. No more narrow hips and concave belly, he said. Instead, it seemed as though I might actually turn into a woman – shock horror – which was most certainly not the desired eternal-girl shape, even amongst provincial GPs.

This noxious attitude goaded me enough to waddle out and buy Susie Orbach's newly published book, *Fat is a Feminist Issue*. Fat and sex, she wrote in 1978, are equally central in the lives of women, and:

> in the United States 50 per cent of women were estimated to be overweight. Every women's magazine has a diet column. Diet doctors and clinics flourish. The names of diet foods are now part of our general vocabulary. Physical fitness and beauty are every woman's goals. While this preoccupation with fat and food has become so common that we tend to

take it for granted, being fat, feeling fat and the compulsion to overeat are, in fact, serious and painful experiences for the women involved.

Not much has changed, has it? During the last century our preoccupation with losing weight has increased, even becoming, according to some psychiatrists, a national neurosis. We have a common aversion to fat – an aesthetic distaste, not to be confused with concerns over obesity and health, though the two are often conflated – and we have a multimillion-pound slimming industry to go with it. Our culture has an endless array of celebrities for us to gawp at: archetypal silent, skinny, schoolgirl-women and waif-boys, eminently enviable and emulated by all groups and ages. They are constantly reported to be on weight-loss diets or to be eating 'healthily' (and, we're reassured, the steak and chips eaten at the press lunch is the ultra-thin star's genuine everyday diet). The present glut of self-loathing, shame and pointless misery of trying and failing to be the ideal creature of our society's desire needs re-thinking. We must rebel against the futility of the present Western beauty norm by exploring and exposing the long and dirty history of body-shaping and dieting so that we can make the crucial shift away from this slavery towards a diet that is healthy both physiologically and psychologically. Dieting is a process on which one embarks laden with emotion, often in an attitude of self-flagellation, and the whole enterprise is salted with the potential for failure.

Yet we all diet sometimes and most of us are adept at the self-delusion which is, let's be honest, necessary for embarking on a fast, and perhaps excessive, weight-loss regimen. The process is like being in love, it provokes the same feelings: an unforgiving and complex mix of the physical sensations and mental tortures of wanting. There you are, dieting, yearning for something. Food is the immediate desire, and thinness the more remote but possibly achievable goal; you are desperate for two things that are out of immediate reach. You dwell obsessively on the object of your love, running over and over it in your mind, discussing it endlessly with others, worrying at it and fantasising about it. It's a sensation not unlike romantic love: it's appetite, perhaps an unquenchable one, a ravenous one. It's not just your body, of course, but your mind too – and that's the bit that really needs to change. We are a culture in pursuit of the perfect diet and the perfect body, and there are a lot of unhappy and insecure people around to prove it.

In fact, a recent survey of 5,000 people found that more than 60 per cent of women in relationships feel decidedly uncomfortable eating in front of their partners. Up to 40 per cent of women feel like they are always dieting or are constantly concerned about their weight; 25 per cent of them thought about food every thirty minutes but just 10 per cent thought about sex as often (men are said to think about sex much more frequently, with 36 per cent fantasising every half an hour). Some women were also concerned with dieting when eating out, choosing low calorie foods in restaurants instead of what they really wanted, and many admitted eating junk food in secret and then lying about it. Lies and insecurities are the bread and butter of much of the popular dieting and body-shape commentary and advice. What are we to make, for example, of the ecstatic coverage of the Duchess of Cambridge's pre-wedding diet and her dramatic dress-size drop? This is especially troubling given how often we've been told that Princess Diana's bulimia began in the lead up to her wedding. Must women have no scary female flesh at all? Is even a little fat so unacceptable? Kate Middleton's mother, we are told, dropped two dress sizes on the Dukan diet and recent research has argued that daughters mimic their mother's dieting and eating habits, and that a mother's dieting history is her daughter's dieting future.

With as many as one-third of all men and women in the Western world thought to be overweight and, unsurprisingly, twice that number believing themselves to be so, the diet industry is sitting pretty. In America alone, an astonishing $40 billion a year is spent on slimming and there truly is something for everyone. You can try the Cabbage Soup diet, or the Grapefruit diet, the Three-day diet, the One-day diet, the Scarsdale diet, the Zone diet, the South Beach diet, the F-Plan diet, the GI diet, the Atkins, the Dukan, the MacDougall Plan, the Prism, the Pritikin, the Hay, the Hollywood, the Russian Air Force diet, the Better Sex diet, the Blood Type diet, the Açai Berry diet, the Hallelujah diet, caveman diets, detoxifying diets, hypno-diets, negative calorie, food-combining diets, the magic-bullet diets, even eating naked in front of the mirror … We are bombarded via technology, too, from the self-improvement vinyl record series of the 1960s, such as Edward L. Baron's 'Reduce Through Listening' which 'helps you develop a dislike for fattening foods', to the iPhone apps of today. Always in your pocket, your iPhone can keep track of your food intake and calorie consumption. You can whip it out whenever a morsel of food threatens you or you feel like scoffing something inappropriate. You can set yourself goals, record your every bite, diligently follow your own progress and see how much weight you're losing or gaining, get instant internet help and tie-ins with proprietary diet regimens, some free, some not, and be swamped by advertising. There are apps that can scan product bar codes and automatically download the calorie count into a daily planner. You can check on yourself in the most obsessive way. We are, it seems, caught in panic-diet mode, trying anything, feeling the pressure from all sides and the misery on the inside.

Fat people have always provoked embarrassment, and even bullying, both individually and commercially, but successful weight loss has to begin with a personal decision. And who ever makes a good decision under pressure? Fat-acceptance activists argue that body fat is not the problem but that what counts is how it is presented in our culture. Influential women such as the singer Beth Ditto intend, according to Germaine Greer, to force acceptance of their body type (Ditto is about 5 ft tall and 15 stone) and so challenge the conventional imagery of women. A good move – as long as the health risks that are associated with being excessively overweight are also publicised. But it will still be an uphill struggle when there is big money to be made and a seemingly bottomless pit of private insecurities to be excavated.

When science tells us that our body's basic instinct to store calories is stronger than our sexual instinct, you know that dieting is a much more complex process than it might seem. Now is the time to ditch the torments – the mad fad diets, slimming drugs and artificial manipulations – needed to squeeze and force ourselves into an unattainable norm of perfection that robs us of our dignity, our cash and our health. Health and contentment are the aims but there's no money in these for the diet industry. Fat is a synonym for the worthless, the slow, the inert, the unattractive, the weak, the poor and the stupid. We have to scrutinise the way in which our culture is exploiting fat at the same time as it castigates it, how we in the West are caught between attractively packaged fast foods and anxiety-inducing diets within a culture that understands fat as bad. The whole diet industry has invested in magical thinking and novelty, it is in the lucrative business of selling hope to the miserable and desperate and creating a vicious circle of hopelessness. It uses its guile to lure us into the Next Big Idea, one that will inevitably involve monstrously detailed instructions, eating food you don't recognise, or some drug or magic bracelet accessory, or mechanical device. And of course most of these come with pricey built-in failure rates that pave the way for the Next, Next Big Idea.

Greed and profit drive the diet market, and complicated

diet plans and paraphernalia just distract the mind from what's required and from the ordinary and inescapable fact that you have to make sensible choices and stick to them. The more difficult a diet is to work out and follow, the more likely the dieter is to give up – and try something else. This reinforces the feelings of failure and benefits an industry which has a vested interest in making losing weight seem a complicated business. We need to know about eating well, to dismiss the diet fads and gurus so that we can ditch the self-loathing and the shame.

The all-consuming story of dieting began in barely recorded pre-history but it really took off some two thousand years ago when the Greeks, who knew for a fact that carrying too much fat is bad for you, developed a fundamentally sound way of addressing it – which is still relevant to us today.

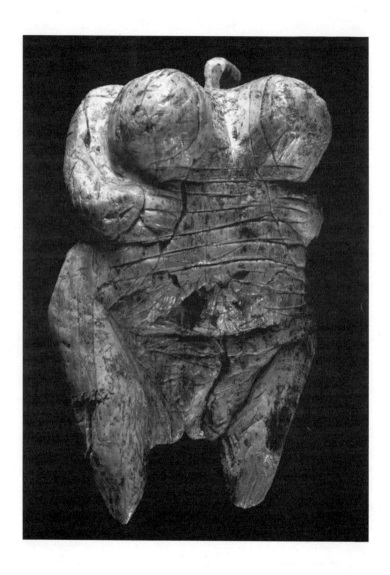

2. The voluptuous and sexually charged Hohle Fels Venus, a tiny female figurine carved from mammoth ivory and unearthed in Germany in 2008 is at least 35,000 years old. She is the earliest depiction we have of the human form, her body is short and squat with huge breasts and a waist that is slightly narrower than her broad shoulders and wide hips. Undeniably excessively curvaceous, she shows that fat is not just a modern phenomenon.

2

The Origin of the Diet

Agayns glotonye is the remedie abstinence

Chaucer

FAT PEOPLE ARE NOTHING NEW. Fat women, especially, have appeared in art and artefacts across the centuries: one of the earliest found examples of figurative art and a representation of an immensely fat woman is the Hohle Fels Venus. Dug up not long ago in Germany, the Venus is a carved mammoth ivory figurine estimated to be about 35,000 years old. There are even earlier hominid figures that could be said to represent obesity: it is thought that the Venus of Berekhat Ram, which was discovered in the Golan Heights, could date from sometime between 230,000 and 500,000 BC; and the Venus of Tan-Tan, from Morocco, is also said to be a relic of this period. If this is so, then neither piece would have been the work of Homo sapiens, but of Homo erectus. The question is whether the large breasts and rolls of fat on the bellies and thighs of the figurines reveal the shape some women actually were, or whether they are stylised, symbolic forms, perhaps of fertile, pregnant or lactating women or, even, it has been suggested, interestingly in the light of our present-day Western obsession with thinness, of ancient pornography.

Some anthropologists and medics say that these prehistoric artefacts are too few and far between to argue that there has always been a natural and apparently widespread propensity to become very fat, while others believe that they are not at all a rare or surprising phenomenon. As long ago as 1939, R. Hautin wrote his essay, *A Historical Framework for the Development of Ideas About Obesity* agreeing with the latter suggestion, saying that, 'the women immortalized in stone age sculpture were fat; there is no other word for it. Obesity was already a fact of life for palaeolithic man – or at least for palaeolithic women.' Images of obesity have recurred over the ages. It is possible that fatness became more common as agricultural settlements began to take over from hunter-gatherer tribes some 12,000 years ago. Queen Hatchepsut, who became pharaoh in Egypt in around 1479 BC and who is regarded as one of the most successful rulers, might have been particularly fat as evidence of 'pendulous breasts' was found in her mummified remains and a contemporary wall painting shows her as, without doubt, a very big woman.

The insults that are often used against fat people – the secret, and often not so secret, moral and physical judgements that we all make – also have ancient and deeply tenacious roots. The old disease of polysarcia, the pathological condition of too much flesh, was thought to indicate a lazy, phlegmatic, stupid person who just could not control themselves. Those reprobates, 'who are uncommonly fat', would also, according to the ancient Greeks, 'die more quickly than the lean'. Like our modern medical profession, however, the ancients were no strangers to contradiction, and they also believed that, 'in all maladies, those who are fat about the belly do best; it is bad to be thin and wasted there'.

The Greek word *diaita*, from which our word 'diet' derives, described a whole way of life rather than referring to a narrow, weight-loss regimen. It provided an all-round mental and physical way to health, basic to one's very existence and success. Greek and Roman physicians knew that how the body functioned was largely dependent on what an individual ate, and that different foods could affect people in different ways. The whole foundation of Western medical science relied on *diatetica*, the fundamental healing therapy of a regimen of certain foods. Being too fat, or too thin, was therefore seen as a sure sign of an unhealthy body, an imbalance of its essential 'humours' (of which there were four: black bile, yellow bile, blood and phlegm). Fat women, for example, were said to find it difficult to conceive, and recent medical studies have confirmed this. Fat men were believed more likely to die earlier, and modern cardiological science has again shown this to be true.

The Greek philosopher and physician Hippocrates (c.460–370 BC) relied on experience and philosophy to discern the truth about human frailties and was as uncompromising about our bodies as he was rational about his prescriptions. His *Corpus Hippocraticum* recommends the observation of nature and the study of evidence in the search for causes of disease. There were two main areas to study: alimentation (the nourishment of life) and the environment we inhabit. Hippocrates understood that the underlying principles of health were food and exercise, or work, and that a high food intake meant that a lot of hard work was needed for it to be properly assimilated. A failure to balance an excess of either would upset the body's metabolism and disease would surely follow. 'Man,' he wrote, 'cannot live healthily on food without a certain amount of exercise.' Walking was considered a natural exercise and, even though it 'partakes somewhat of the violent kind', if you did it after eating it would prevent the accumulation of abdominal fat, especially if you walked extra fast. More 'violent' exercise, including running long distances and gradually increasing your exertions, helped to burn off excess food in the body and was thought 'suitable for people who eat too much', along with the 'induction of vomiting' which he considered especially beneficial.

Still, Hippocrates' fundamental premise was right. He knew that it was impossible to prescribe a rigorously perfect regimen for all, one in which the amount of food would exactly counterbalance the amount of exercise in every individual case. People's constitutions were not all alike, and individual requirements varied according to age, climate, season, and so on. Food, too, was very variable, that is, 'there are different varieties of cheese, different varieties of wine and of all other foods in the composition of our daily intake'. Despite these varieties any sudden change in one's regimen was to be carefully avoided, and the amount of food and exercise taken had to be reduced gradually, week by week. In the summer, breakfasts ought be 'light and food not excessive … as much drink as possible must be taken during meals but not in between. Suitable vegetables, cooked or raw, must be had in abundance.' Furthermore, this being a way-of-life diet, baths should be taken lukewarm and sexual intercourse avoided whenever possible.

He observed that people who ate too much presented with all sorts of symptoms: at first they frequently fell into a prolonged and pleasant sleep at night, and even for short intervals during the day, but the fatter they got the worse their sleep became until it was 'less agreeable, more disturbed and in their dreams they struggle.' Their heavy, uncomfortable fullness, or plethoric state, produced aches and pains over part or all of the body as well as a feeling of utter fatigue which made the sufferer believe that he or she was really tired. The danger was that they would try to relieve these feelings with rest and a good feeding but this would soon lead to further ill health. Others were recorded as suffering from flatulence because they were not absorbing the excess food, and a high temperature may be present along with constipation because the bowels failed to work properly 'in proportion to the food taken'. Hippocrates' patients were often found to vomit up their food the following day, undigested, with acid eructations producing 'a burning sensation up the throat and even into the nostrils', and they had bad complexions and rotten headaches. And, as for having sex, while one might experience a sense of immediate relief, beware, for the feelings of heaviness will be worse later on: 'The danger is great.'

What to do? For obese people with a laxity of muscle and red complexions, Hippocrates recommended dry food to help with their moist constitution but, in general, a diet of light and emollient (soothing or softening) foods was needed to assist with the evacuation of the bowel, 'thus enabling the lower part to relieve the congestion of the upper'. Slow running, considerable morning walks, and even wrestling were to be actively encouraged. The very fat, especially 'those desiring to lose weight', were told to indulge in a spot of hard work and to eat while still panting from their efforts. Their meals were to be prepared with sesame or seasoning and other similar substances, and be of a fatty nature so that they would feel as full as possible on very little food. They should, moreover, eat just one main meal a day and take only wine with it, diluted and slightly cold. Breakfast should never be missed, and after breakfast one could perhaps have a bit of a sleep and, later in the day, one of those walks. In fact, they should walk naked for as long as possible and then sleep on a hard bed. Every morning, for the following six days, the walks and exercises should be gradually increased until, on the seventh day, a full meal was to be followed by vomiting. Vomiting, bathing and anointing were good (as long as the bath was only lukewarm), and would do instead of all the sloth-inducing sex you weren't allowed to have. And so on, all over again, for a four-week period.

To us, this advice seems mixed, some sensible, some inadvisable if not dangerous, but it would all have made sense at the time, based as it was on contemporary knowledge and practices. Induced vomiting, for example, which might horrify us today, was popular and almost an art form, as the following attests: 'fat individuals should vomit in the middle of the day, after a running or marching exercise and before taking any food. The emetic may be half a cup of hyssop (0.15 litre) ground with three litres of water, to which vinegar and salt is added to render the drink as agreeable as possible. The whole of it is to be taken beginning with a small and gradually increasing quantity.' If enemas were prescribed for the obese they had to be thin and salty, and sea water was best of all. Vinegar was a great favourite in the treatment of excessive fat, its properties being regarded as dry and warm and so antithetical to fat bodies which were considered moist and cool.

In the classical world, what foods you ate, and how much, played an important role in ethical teachings and philosophical and political thinking, and centred on ideas of luxury and corruption. Food was for sustenance alone and to overindulge was morally and physically bad for you. Everyone knew that luxury would excite the passions which, once aroused, could result in an undignified slide into moral and physical degradation. To Socrates (469–399 BC) the pleasures and comforts of a civilised diet generated increasing demands for luxuries, not only for palatable delicacies but for scent and cosmetics, mistresses, the fine arts of painting and embroidery, for gold and for ivory: a really slippery slope. All these luxuries and the greed that went with them would, he cautioned, lead inevitably to wars and unjust societies. If appetite should outstrip self-control then it was not just your body that would suffer, your very soul was in danger, and civilisation would wither.

Cravings for strong foods, full of heat, were thought to give rise to sexual promiscuity, a social as well as personal danger, and literature on food began to record astonishing descriptions of feasts, of gluttony and lechery. Stories of the eating, drinking and sexual proclivities of well-known members of society abounded and could bolster or destroy reputations, whether they were based in truth or not and this has continued throughout history.

The Greek Sicilian chef, Archestratus of Gela, wrote a poem, *Hedypatheia* (Pleasant Living), in the fourth century BC, in praise of the life of luxury, and was mentioned along with twenty other writers on food and cooking, by the Greek gourmet Athenaeus who wrote the *Deipnosophistae* (The Learned Banquet), a long, third-century AD account of the luxuries associated with dining. These works on eating and drinking revealed attitudes, opinions and, not least, contemporary emotions involved with food. They laid emphasis on simplicity and abstention and so were concerned with the moral aspects of cooking and eating as well. Works such as Petronius's *Satyricon*, a first-century Roman 'novel', parodied sensual culinary excesses in its description of a feast given by the character Trimalchio. Trimalchio is an ex-slave made good, and his vulgar, flamboyant indulgences at the table end with his household and guests acting out his own funeral. Plutarch, a Greek historian writing at around the same time, discussed the problem of obesity and health, saying that 'thin people are generally the most healthy' and drawing the conclusion that 'we should not therefore indulge our appetites with delicacies or high living, for fear of growing corpulent'. He described the body as 'a ship which must not be overloaded', and wrote that a good doctor was one who used diet rather than drugs or the knife. Scribonius Largus, first-century court physician to the Roman emperor Claudius, agreed, and summed up the stages of medical cure as, first and foremost, diet, then drugs, and lastly cautery or surgery. A good and moderate diet – no extremes or faddish behaviour – was by far the most important and successful way of treating disease. Caution and moderation were everything.

If diet was your route to health it was also, if abused, the way to disease and death. This meant that, in this period, responsibility lay with the individual who had it in his or her power to control their physical and mental state. Choosing how one lived was therefore a moral question; one had a duty to oneself but also to society. This sat well with the contemporary Stoic view which, simply put, stated that virtue, endurance and self-sufficiency would lead to truth, health and happiness. Moderation and balance were essential in all things, including one's diet, a philosophy that placed the ordinary business of eating within the moral order.

The extremely influential, second-century Greek physician Galen (c. 130–c. 200 BC), a follower of Hippocrates, produced *On the Power of Foods*, which contained an all-round explanation of the dietary habits of the Roman Empire. Good doctors, he thought, should also be good cooks and he often included recipes in his works. Recounting one of the earliest known case studies of treatment for obesity, Galen wrote that he had 'reduced a huge fat fellow to a moderate size in a short time, by making him run every morning until he fell into a profuse sweat; I then had him rubbed hard, and put into a warm bath ... Some hours after, I permitted him to eat freely of food, which afforded but little nourishment; and lastly, set him to some work.' He also cited the case of one Nicomachus of Smyrna, who was so huge that he couldn't even get up from his bed. Other commentators noted the enormous size a Roman senator had achieved, so big that he was only able to walk when two of his slaves carried his belly for him, and another, an Egyptian pharaoh whose middle was wider than the span of his slave's outstretched arms. Dionysius of Heraclea was famous for his gargantuan appetite, and got so fat that he, too, could barely move or be moved. He suffered, it is thought, from either apnea or narcolepsy so that he had to have people around him to prick his flesh with needles should he fall asleep on his throne. A contemporary poet recorded that Dionysius said he wanted to die 'on my back, lying on my many rolls of fat, scarcely uttering a word, taking laboured breaths, and eating my fill', a death of luxurious excess and satiation. He died at fifty-five, an object of great and general fascination because of his enormous body.

Early ascetics such as Saint Anthony, who, at the end of the third century, went off to live the solitary life in the desert east of the Nile, also attracted intense contemporary attention and wonderment for quite different reasons. Their heroic abstinence and starved bodies were often the subject of exaggerated glorification. The manner in which ascetics chose to starve their bodies is unclear, but much of the surviving literature suggests a destructive dualism, a real hostility to their physical selves. This may have been in part directed against sexual desire but was more generally an aversion to the demands the body made upon the soul, demands that were feared as demonic distractions from the focus on God. Food and eating, as perfect vehicles for ritual, are central to most religions, often differentiating one sect or denomination from another.

As the anthropologist Meyer Fortes puts it, it is not so much that food is good to eat as that it is good to forbid, and Mary Douglas, the British anthropologist, has argued that food is not only a metaphor or vehicle of communication but a physical event and so a powerful and symbolic means of denial. Eating habits have social and moral components and reveal all sorts of messages about human needs, about the separation of spirit and flesh, about the physical functions of ingestion, excretion and corruption, and the guarding of orifices. Using prayer to banish fat has a long history, from St Augustine of Hippo in the third century AD to Deborah Pierce in 1960, author of *I Prayed Myself*

Slim. These modern Christian weight-loss plans are heavy on the ambiguity, however, because the body is both an obstacle to spiritual growth and a tool for cultivating that growth – both eating and fasting have the same potential for sin or salvation. Such conflicting attitudes have a profound influence on people's relationships with food and their bodies.

The ancient way to true asceticism was through 'never giving the self its fill of bread, nor water, nor sleep, and tormenting oneself with appetite for these things, not feelings of lust'. Porphyry's *Life of Plotinus*, a third-century neo-Platonist philosopher, said of his subject that he 'appeared ashamed of being in the body'. Philostratus's third-century *Life of Apollonius of Tyana* describes a regimen of five years' silence, celibacy, refusal to wear clothes and shoes made from animal products, or to eat any foods bar dried fruit and vegetables, with the result that, 'even when young and vigorous he mastered the body and was in control of his passions'. The Egyptian hermit Dorotheus said, when asked about his extreme austerities, 'It [the body] kills me, so I kill it.' Theodore of Skyeon, in sixth-century Anatolia, was said to have 'nobly mortified his body, keeping it under and wearing it down, as though it were some alien thing which warred against the soul'. As a philosophical idea, self-control to whatever degree stretches as far back as Socrates and was a continuing theme through ancient philosophy, from the Stoic view that true humanity lies in controlling oneself and exercising moderation in the face of the powerful desires for food, drink and sex, to the neo-Pythagorean concept of bodily austerity as a means to spiritual insight. To philosophers, physicians and the common man alike, the physical self was an object of deservedly anxious attention, and some disgust. The human body required constant control to keep it in balance, to dry it and to achieve and maintain continence, a difficult and continuous task best done through diet.

Early Christian ascetics, similarly, viewed the body as something apart, to be approached only with a deep sense of detached mistrust, as something to be dominated, something seen to be denied. This enactment of abstinence was almost theatrical in nature, a drama displayed before a captivated audience. As the church became established, one of the ways in which temptation and greed, those intense and selfish desires, were written on the body was in fat, obvious and showy. The ideal, slender, exiguous body had always been deemed divine and in stark contrast to the mortal and sinful body grown large and wanton in flesh.

Even St Augustine of Hippo struggled daily with his desire to eat and drink, far more than he ever did with his feelings of sexual lust. His greediness was 'not an evil which I can decide once and for all to repudiate and never to embrace again, as I was able to do with fornication'. Even regarding his food as a form of medicine, as was common, he still felt sure that the 'snare of concupiscence' awaited him. The very process of passing from the discomfort of hunger to the comfort of satiation was 'a pleasure and there is no other means of satisfying hunger except the one'. So, caught in a cleft stick, he felt himself obliged to eat, even though he knew he would suffer for it.

Gluttony, far more so than the six other deadly sins, was a visible sin, embodied in opulent flesh, an outward sign of a soul sold to another God. This is Pauline philosophy: all humans are damned for their flesh. Women, being weak and pathologically corrupt creatures, were particularly susceptible to temptation and the early church fathers were especially obsessed with what they did with their bodies. When comparisons are made now between the early fasting saints and modern excessive dieting, the suggestion is that unusually high numbers of young female deaths in the thirteenth century might have been a response to Christian teaching, and it does not seem too far-fetched an argument. In the late 1970s and 1980s fundamentalist Christian groups in America were producing books which promoted rigorous weight loss for women.

Habitual overeating has traditionally been regarded with the utmost distaste, and Christian notions of gluttony included not just gross indulgence, but connoisseurship. In the sixth century, Pope Gregory the Great had identified several different kinds of gluttony, such as:

eating too much (*nimis*)
eating with unbecoming eagerness (*ardenter*)
eating wildly (*forente*)
not waiting until decent mealtimes (*praepropere*)
enjoying food that was too expensive (*laute*)
and being too picky (*studiose*)

All these eating behaviours were regarded as equally sinful. Excessive picky daintiness encompassed both fussing over the preparation of food and medical or hypochondriacal concerns with it. Lust and gluttony, two of the Catholic deadly sins, were thought to complement and encourage each other, being quintessentially physical sins as opposed to the mental transgressions of pride or envy. St Thomas Aquinas was an enormously fat Catholic priest and philosopher who was so big by the time he died that his pall-bearers had trouble fitting him into his grave. In the thirteenth century he was preaching right-mindedness, part of which was the established idea that greed and gluttony were matters of the soul. If you happened to be fat, as he was, your body spoke volumes about your struggle with spiritual health. With a troubled eye on the hereafter Aquinas wrote: 'Let us not give our minds to delights but to what is the end of delights. Here on earth it is excrement and obesity, hereafter it is fire and the worm.' So early Christian attitudes to food were already complicated, involving temptation, sin and punitive redemption. They borrowed much from the classical Greek theory of *diatetica*, linked, as the Christian approach was, to duty and morality, but obscured it, just as it is obscured today by novelty, dissatisfaction and a fixation with celebrity culture. But *diatetica* is a deeply sensible plan for living and eating that, though relevant today, has been largely discarded in favour of the faster and more superficial approaches that have their roots in popular early modern diet regimens.

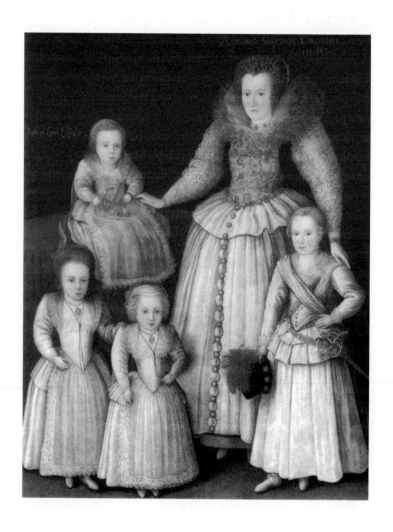

3. Body-shapes are dictated by fashion and are nothing new. Corsetry has been popular for hundreds of years and these restrictive garments were worn by children as well as adults as shown above in the portrait of the Countess of Leicester and her children (1596). Originally made of metal, horn and whalebone with seams, gores, buttons and lacing, corsets drew in waists and bellies even during times of bad harvests and food scarcity. The bad breath and over-lapping ribs which were said to result from the luxurious vanity of corset-wearing were still a problem three-hundred years later.

3

Luxury and Sloth

TODAY, THERE IS ALWAYS A NEW dieting manual on the best-seller lists, many of which promote unsustainable diets or re-hashes of previous fads, often endorsed by a celebrity whose unattainably slim body betrays hours of work and a lot of cash investment. But it wasn't always like this. Medieval and early modern books on food and eating were still based on sound classical diet ideas, although some revealed anxieties about the 'ideal body'. One of the earliest ever regimens specifically for weight loss was devised for those who did not match up to this 'beauty of the form of the body', meaning those who suffered from 'undue thinness and fatness'. The eleventh-century plan, prescribed by Avicenna, a Persian physician and philosopher, advises the fat and unhealthy to eat only bulky food with little nutrition in it and then to help it move through their bodies as quickly as possible with the aid of laxatives and exercise. Avicenna's weight-loss answer is still extremely popular nearly a thousand years later though still no more successful as a long-term solution.

The first 'modern' best-seller, the cosmopolitan and popular fifteenth-century *De honesta voluptate et valetudine*, by

Bartolomeo Sacchi (Il Platina) (1421–81) attempted to bring pleasure (*voluptate*) and health (*valetudine*) together. Platina was a humanist writer who supplemented recipes borrowed from other works with some of Galen's medical advice to produce a practical cookery book in an attempt to balance dietetics (the science of eating for good health) with gastronomy (a philosophy of eating well for pleasure and cultural refinement). The book got caught up in the culture-changing development of the printing press revolution and so was available to a much wider readership than any before. It was first published in Rome in 1470, in Florence and Venice in 1472, and later in Germany before it ran through several subsequent editions. By 1505 it had been translated and adapted into French as *Le Platine en françoys* and became one of most important works on diet and eating in early modern Europe. In his eighth book, Platina concentrated on condiments, spices and the enhancement of flavour and, after a list of more than sixty condiments one could use, he noted that 'Nothing given to us to eat is so flavourless that sugar does not season it.' This advice was qualified, however, with a warning to his readers not to use spices and the like for 'luxury, lust and intemperance'. Following acknowledged historic wisdom, he regarded these vices as prevalent in Rome and other Italian cities where the people's appetites were so jaded that they could only be stimulated by artificial means (and also where many of them were dangerously fat).

Post-Renaissance food writing was all about a proper understanding of how plain, wholesome food could nourish the body. The prevailing belief was that a good diet would lead to healthier lives for all and thus a happier and more prosperous society. Xenophon's *Of Household*, published in Latin in 1508 and reissued five times by 1526, addressed the gentry and wealthier classes who aspired to a simple and satisfying home-produced diet to counter their hankerings for more exotic and unhealthy items, in a way that is reminiscent of the middle-class organic movement of today. The less well-off, who needed stamina for physical work, were already eating this good diet of bean and cereal pottage, bread, dumplings, puddings and pies and didn't have access to large quantities of meat and other food luxuries.

The dietetic rationale of books such as Thomas Elyot's *Castel of Helth* (1534), Andrew Boorde's *Compendyous Regyment of a Dyetry of Health* (1542), William Vaughan's *Naturall and Artificial Directions for Health* (1602) and Thomas Moffett's *Health's Improvement* (1655) expressly conveyed this civic ideal and were concerned with problems of excessive consumption. They recommended a diet not far removed from peasant food; moderation and frugality were the watchwords. Yet there was a contradiction between this directive and the sometimes lavish efforts that went into the preparation of particular dishes.

Sir Thomas Elyot published *Castel of Helth* as a medical work with opinions on diet. Elyot was a well-travelled diplomat and scholar, an intimate of Wolsey and Thomas Cromwell, and a supporter of humanist ideas concerning the education of women (his *The Defence of Good Women* was published in 1540). His book was derided by his peers but appreciated by the general public, and it speedily went through seventeen editions. Like Hippocrates before him, Elyot understood the healthy human body as resting on the balance between the four principle humours (Greek medical ideas were adhered to until well into the eighteenth century). Different foods generated different humours, and one learned by experience what foods suited one's body: fish was inferior to meat because it thinned the blood; butter was nourishing; cheese was the enemy of the stomach; turnips were thought to enhance virility and 'augment the seed of man'; fruit could be dangerous as it brought on ill-humours which might rise to putrefying fevers if eaten continually; alcohol made one sickly (Cornish people were strong and healthy because they drank only water); and a mixture of different meats at one meal was very bad for the constitution. Elyot followed classical writers on the merits of coleworts and cabbages as medicines against all diseases, and was prejudiced against spices which he considered were brought to England only 'to content the insatiableness of wanton appetites'. He concluded that gluttony was an abuse rife in the kingdom. Again, simplicity and restraint were the thing.

Temperate eating was also advised by one of Elyot's contemporaries, the physician Andrew Boorde (c. 1490–1549). As a young man, Boorde had been a Carthusian monk but, in 1521, he 'dispensed of religion' in favour of medicine and was always practical in his advice. He, too, condemned gluttony, saying that two meals a day should be quite enough for those leading a gentle, sedentary life, while three meals a day were necessary for people whose work was more physically demanding. In contradistinction to Elyot, Boorde recorded that the Cornish drank an ale so vile, white and thick that it looked and tasted as though pigs had wrestled in it.

Disapproval and disgust were evident in the writings of these powerful and educated men, many of whom were involved in court politics. Henry VIII's eating habits (his insatiably greedy appetite, particularly for globe artichokes, was well known) and anxieties over his fat, ungainly body and generally unhealthy state drew increasing public notice as he aged. The politician, John Hales (c. 1516–71), MP for Preston, was extremely worried about gluttony, claiming that more men died from overeating than ever had from the sword or plague – a pretty eye-catching claim in the sixteenth century. Following classical and contemporary advice he advised his readers to accustom themselves to simple foods so that they would be ready to swallow them easily whenever they were sick, but he argued, too, that eating strange and dainty meats when one was not hungry would stir up trouble and dissension in the nation. Thomas Cogan's *Haven of Health* (1584) was written for boys in Protestant England and urged personal bodily self-restraint and management especially in spheres of diet and sexual conduct. This was the basis of the nation's health – physical and moral, spiritual and societal. To maintain a 'meane and temperate dyet, in the feare of God' was a spiritual matter with wide-ranging consequences. Food and politics were irredeemably linked, and Hales had advocated good health rather than corrupt wealth. The mid-sixteenth century was a difficult time of poor harvests and dearth when food prices rose sharply, and though Hales exhorted men to 'make no sedition in the Commonwealth', he was still blamed for whipping up public disturbances. He had based his arguments on those of Plutarch and called for 'moderate and mean fare' for his fellow statesmen and peasants alike. This mean fare was a 'sodden' pottage, frumenty (a sort of spiced porridge), bread sops and greenstuffs, usually washed down with water. The availability of foods, and the act of eating, represented a fragile dependence on an insecure world of dearth and possible starvation. This anxiety would surface after the world wars of the twentieth century, as we shall see.

In the mid-seventeenth century, hunger arising from poor harvests, and the attendant political manoeuvring, encouraged the Royal Society to explore the idea of hunger-suppressing foods. This was an early subject for the men of the Royal Society, an organisation founded in 1660 to discuss the new philosophy of knowledge through observation and experiment. In 1662 members were urged to support the planting of potatoes, and Robert Boyle, influential founding member and father of modern experimental methods, promised to supply some for trial by his fellows. In the early 1680s in Scotland there was renewed interest in classical writers such as Pliny who had written on hunger-suppressing foods used in the ancient world as well as in similar references made in the literature of ancient Britons and Highlanders. Experiments were conducted using plants such as heath pea or caremyle, otherwise known as bitter vetch (Lathyrus linifolius), colloquially known in Scotland as 'knappers'. Dr James Fraser, who became Secretary of the Chelsea Royal Hospital, experimented on himself with doses of caremyle, which he likened to liquorice, and found he could comfortably go without food for sixty-six hours. Interest grew and was encouraged at the highest level by Charles II and his court. Sir Robert Sibbald, co-founder of the Royal College of Physicians of Edinburgh and of the Botanic Garden, published a treatise in 1699 entitled *Provision for the Poor in Time of Dearth and Scarcity*, where there is an 'Account of such Food as may easily be Gotten when Corns are Scarce and Unfit for Use'.

Alongside these efforts at assuaging the hunger that arose from lack were developments in the eating habits of the better-off. At the start of the seventeenth century, when world exploration was in full swing, new foods had begun to reach the British Isles and were beginning to change some people's diets as well as their attitudes to different tastes and textures. The range of available foods broadened, foreign influences became more apparent, and certain food fashions that took off among the well-to-do filtered down through the layers of society. Sugar arrived. In bulk. A new era began when honey was usurped as the traditional sweetener and, in London at least, sugar was soon regarded as the healthier option. It had made an early appearance in Holinshed's *Chronicles* in around 1577 when sugarbread was roundly scorned as a new and outlandish confection, a foolish conceit provided by comfit-makers (a profession first recorded in 1594) and indulged in by the gentry. Comfit-makers coated sweetmeats and fruits in sugar, producing a time-consuming and expensive food for the urban rich. The records of the Reynell family, who lived in rural Devon, reveal that their sugar consumption had increased from twenty-four pounds in 1629 to forty pounds in 1631. By 1676, books such as *Rules for Health* were recommending a weighing chair that could measure the weight of a diner after his meal and act as a guide for precise food intake; other commentators, such as Leonardo Lessia, advised weighing food before eating it, a control that did not, however, understand the relationship of particular foods to the accumulation of body fat.

In the seventeenth century, attitudes to the temptations and vanity of Eve (female beauty) were based on practical, philosophical or religious ideals, creating and upholding sex differences. They embraced aesthetics as well as order. The British poet Sir John Harington specified the best of early modern feminine beauty as 'skin, and teeth, must be cleare, bright, and neat [with] large brests, large hips'. The first tailored corsets and metal or whalebone rigid stays were available for the wealthy who wished to live up to Harington's ideal. They very visibly accentuated the shape of the female body, with seams, gores, buttons and lacing adding an erotic dimension to corset-wearing. In 1597, the fourteen-year-old daughter of an English gentleman, a Mr Starkie, was accused of being possessed by the devil having demanded 'a French bodie, not of whalebone, for that is not stiff enough but of horne for that will hold it out, it shall come, to keep in my belly'. The French essayist Michel de Montaigne tells of the famous French surgeon, Ambroise Paré, who had opened up some of these 'pretty women with slender waists' on the dissection table, 'lifted the skin and the flesh, and showed us their ribs which overlapped each other'. To get a slim outline these women would endure any self-inflicted pain, it seemed; they were so tightly tied and bound they suffered 'gashes in their sides, right to the living flesh. Yes, sometimes they even die from it'. John Bulwer, in *The Artificial Changeling* (1653), railed against the corset, too:

Another foolish affection there is in young Virgins, though grown big enough to be wiser, but that they are led blindfold by Custome to a fashion pernicious beyond imagination; who thinking a Slender-Waist a great beauty, strive all that they possibly can by straight-lacing themselves fine enough until they can span their Waste. By which deadly artifice they reduce their Breasts into such streights, that they soon purchase a stinking breath; and while they ignorantly affect an August or narrow Breast, and to that end by strong compulsion shut up their Waists in a Whale-bone prison, or little-ease, they open a door to Consumptions, and a withering rottennesse.

Both the alarm at female vanity (and its consequences) and the concomitant development of interest in new foods, deepened the perceived connections between behaviour, health, medicine and diet. Physicians, alchemists, chemists and intellectuals all joined the debate on the benefits of different rules and standards for what they considered to be healthy regimens. The obvious commercial possibilities began to be exploited as fashionable new diets were concocted, promoted and traded upon. Certain foods and drinks were sold as miracle foods, a trade that took off in the Victorian age and is still going strong. Among the new proprietary foods was William Folkingham's 'panala ala catholica', a medicinal composition – brewed of ale and herbs which were to be infused for three days or more and then drunk cold – that was announced to the public in 1623 in a book of the same name. And in 1653 the Countess of Kent published a recipe book that included new cordial waters, also sometimes called diet drinks, which were all the rage at the time among the fashionable classes.

A diet can be something of an odyssey, which is perhaps why we so often need a guide in the form of a diet book or manual. One of the most successful diet books, *The Art of Living Long* by a Venetian merchant named Luigi Cornaro (1464–1566), is still in print over four hundred and fifty years after it was first published in Padua in 1558. It was an instant success, went through many editions, and was translated into many languages. Contemporaries such as Elyot, Boorde, Vaughan and Markham, concerned with what they perceived to be the problem of excessive eating and drinking, had read Cornaro's 'admirable diet', a diet not far removed from the simple peasant food they all advocated. A 1903 edition of *The Art of Living Long* was still advising its readers to take good heed of Cornaro's work, and recommending the spirit of his approach, if not his life-and-death method, the strictness of which could, as today's neurobehaviourists recognise, sometimes backfire.

Cornaro's story is one of sin and redemption and it begins with a no-holds-barred confession about his first forty years that were spent in dissipated, gluttonous overindulgence. This way of life had deprived him of many of his excellent friends so he employed the best physicians to help him undo the self-inflicted damage before he, too, went to an early grave. Eventually the conclusion was reached that only one thing would save him – a sober and regular life. It was diet or die for Cornaro, so he worked out a personal regimen and saved his own life.

The first rule of Cornaro's diet is to regain self-control. Gluttony, he believed, was not merely a personal sin but also a killer. He saw it as an almost apocalyptic force: it 'kills every year … as great a number as would perish during the time of a most dreadful pestilence, or by the sword or fire of many bloody wars'. Citing the ancients, Galen, Hippocrates, Plato and Cicero, he insisted, with the zeal of a convert, on living a regular life of moderation. All passions had to be restrained if not denied, and one should cease to be a slave to pleasures and appetites because they were nothing but fatal delusions. Taste was one such pleasure. The idea that 'what delights the palate, cannot but be good for the heart' was false, he wrote, and only served the sensualists who would suffer in the long run and provide business for the 'apothecary [who] is perpetually employed in countermining the cook and the vintner'. Physic, or medicine, was, for the most part, nothing but a substitute for the actual weight loss necessities of exercise and temperance.

People should eat little and frugally (today's Calorie Restrictors are Cornaro's direct dieting descendants) he advised, and he recommended a diet consisting of twelve ounces a day in bread, soups, yolks of new-laid eggs, meat, plus about fourteen ounces of wine. For meat he suggested sticking to veal, kid, mutton, partridges, pullets and pigeons, and 'among the sea-fish I choose goldenies, and of the river fish the pike'. His granddaughter later recalled that Cornaro even cut down on this intake as he aged, sometimes restricting himself to just the yolk of an egg for his one daily meal, occasionally making it do for two. If he changed his diet at all he discovered that he became ill and saw this as vindication of the great influence a regular regimen has on a body.

Cornaro's diet had other unexpected effects on his body. Not only had he become thin again, he wrote, but he had regained his masculinity, something he felt he had lost through his vain pursuit of luxury and pleasure – indulgences traditionally seen as feminine. This is a cultural hot potato: fat is soft and feminine, for which read 'weak', not hard like the flesh of a 'real' man. Disentangling these matters – the demarcation of fat as a female sexual attribute, body re-shaping and self-image in relation to others (do you opt for disciplined dieting or Let. Yourself. Go.) – is a complicated exercise. Embarking on a diet is no simple undertaking. For a dieter is not just altering his or her physical body shape: they are altering the shape that they occupy in society and, so doing, are changing what their body says to the rest of the world.

'The first physicians by debauch were made, excess began, and sloths sustained the trade,' wrote the poet John Dryden (1631–1700), acknowledging that medicine has long been up against people's greed and wanton appetite. In his epic poem *Paradise Lost* (1667), John Milton, poet and political activist, advised the rule of 'not too much' if one wanted to avoid disease and misery, and he advanced the idea of gluttony being a feminine vice by blaming Eve and the indulgences of her daughters:

> Some, as thou saw'st, by violent stroke shall die,
> By fire, flood, famine; by intemperance more
> In meats and drinks, which on the Earth shall bring
> Diseases, dire, of which a monstrous crew
> Before thee shall appear, that thou may'st know
> What miseries the inabstinence of Eve
> Shall bring on men.
>
> If thou well observe
> The rule of 'Not too much,' by temperance taught
> In what thou eat'st and drink'st, seeking from thence
> Due nourishment, not gluttonous delight,
> Till many years over thy head return;
> So may'st thou live, till, like ripe fruit, thou drop
> Into thy mother's lap, or be with ease
> Gathered, not harshly plucked, for death mature.

Up until the eighteenth century, the concept of the diet, still largely about healthy eating and living, was discussed and written about by physicians, philosophers, poets and politicians. It embraced morality, control, civic duty, self-awareness and balance. The German philosopher Nietzsche, whose sedentary life had made him fat, read Cornaro's book in the late nineteenth century, and was not impressed: 'The extraordinary slowness of [Cornaro's] metabolism,' he wrote, in *Twilight of the Idols and the Anti-Christ* (1888), 'was the cause of his slender diet … a scholar in our time, with his rapid consumption of nervous energy, would simply destroy himself on Cornaro's diet. *Credo experto* – believe me, I've tried.' But, even if Cornaro's diet didn't work for German nihilists, what had been good for sixteenth-century Italians might perhaps be applied to the nineteenth-century English. According to one of the many editions of *The Art of Living Long*, 'what the noble Cornaro observes of the Italians of his time, may with justice be applied to this nation at present'. The overindulgent orders of Victorian society were 'not contented with a plain bill of fare … we ransack the elements of earth, sea, and air for all sorts of creatures, to gratify our wanton and luxurious appetites … to create a false appetite, we rack the inventions of our cooks, for new sauces and provocatives, to make the superfluous morsel go down with the greater gust'.

Given the evidence of our own time, it would be hard to claim that we are any different now: porridge-flavoured ice cream, extra-sweet white chocolate and salty caviar, a combination of beetroot and green peppercorn jelly with mango and pine purée, are all recent examples of culinary experimentation. In America, celebrity chefs such as Emeril Lagasse, and Ina Garten who hosts the popular show *Barefoot Contessa*, produce rich and extraordinary dishes; and in Britain Heston Blumenthal is said to have 600 dishes in the 'design' process while Nigella Lawson – neither a chef nor professional cook – gives her qualification as 'an eater'. Many of our present attitudes to food – the need for variety, the devil-may-care consumption – are ultimately unsatisfying. Luxurious eating is the counterpoint to crash dieting and neither of these will make us content.

Diatetica was the ancient foundation of Western medical science, the fundamental healing therapy of a management regimen that prescribed particular foods and ways of eating. The ancient idea of diet included weight loss where necessary, but was primarily concerned with all-round mental, physical and social health. Dieting was not merely an issue for the individual driven by dissatisfaction and desire but a matter of wider social significance. If one ate well, and with restraint, one could live well, too; but if one was partial to overindulgence not only would there be consequences for the individual but the wider common good would suffer. This truism of the classical period was relevant in the eighteenth century and remains so today. And we'd do well to replace our tendency to associate diet with fashion and celebrity (the vanity and luxury of which the Greeks warned) with a renewed focus on health and well-being.

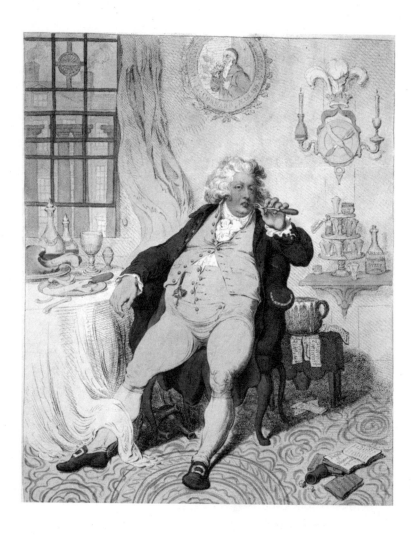

4. The satirical cartoonist Gillray portrays George, Prince of Wales, later Prince Regent and George IV (reigned 1820–30), vulgarly picking his teeth with a table fork after a bout of excessive wining and dining, a picture of greed and waste. Hugely overweight and known as the 'Prince of Whales', he had a reputation for being notoriously dissolute and spendthrift when war, taxation and dearth weighed heavily on the poorer classes. Excess and gluttony, written on his body in flesh, were not just personal failings but moral and political sins, too.

4

Strictly Avoid Frightening Ideas

THE EARLY MEDICAL PROFESSION rather relied on the gross habits of its patients to provide it with a good income. During the eighteenth century, when dissections in the interests of medical research began to increase, physicians such as Giovanni Battista Morgagni made lengthy descriptions of the post-mortems they performed and wrote up detailed case studies of the excessively fat. In older women, Morgagni noted an acquired apple shape, something now known as android obesity, and in older, severely fat men he found a related harden-ing of the arteries. But despite their regard for temperance and all the advice offered to their overweight patients, the physicians themselves sometimes got very fat, too.

George Cheyne (1671–1743), who weighed over 32 stone, was an eminent physician and philosopher from Scotland, a Fellow of the College of Physicians at Edinburgh and a Fellow of the Royal Society. After having settled first in London and later in Bath, he built up a lucrative practice treating the aristocratic, professional, and occasionally neurotic upper classes: 'the nervous disorders being computed to make almost one third of the complaints of the people of condition in England'. A 'Malregimen of Diet' was what, in his mind, accounted for true manias, real lunacy and a disordered brain.

Cheyne recognised the vital connection between his mental state and his ballooning body size. During his early years in London his weight increased dramatically and he was reduced to a death-obsessed anxiety. 'Upon my coming to London,' he wrote, 'I all of a sudden changed my whole manner of living; I found the bussle, companions, the younger gentry and free-livers, to be the most easy of access, and most quickly susceptible of friend-ship and acquaintance, nothing being necessary for that purpose but to be able to eat lustily, and swallow down much liquor.' His intimate and confessional manner informed the advice he gave to others, and he urged his patients to self-maintenance and abstinence as he attributed his own illnesses to conspicuous over-indulgence. Struggling constantly with his weight and accompa-nying depression, he believed that one should attempt to tame one's passions and appetites through diet and God – Cheyne, apparently, was usually to be found in coffeehouses and taverns, with 'free-livers' and 'bottle-companions', talking about naked faith and pure love, a divided man constantly trying to reconcile his physical and mental self. He published several very successful works, including his *Essay on Gout* (1720), an *Essay on Health and Long Life* (1724) which ran to nine editions in his lifetime and was translated into several European languages, and *The English Malady* (1733), a work on melancholy and the difficult relation-ship between the spirit and the flesh. The treatments he recom-mended were soundly based on temperance and vegetarianism, and among his friends and patients he counted the most noted philosophers and writers of his day, including David Hume, Samuel Richardson, Samuel Johnson, John Wesley, Alexander Pope, the Earl of Huntingdon and the Duke of Roxburghe. The idea of a morbidly fat physician advising on dietary matters seems not to have caused them too much food for thought.

Cheyne's books recommend a pure and plain diet, uncorrupted and reasonable. One needed nothing, he argued, but good sense, solid virtue and true Christian courage to fight prejudice and appetite. It was hard to make a stand against rich and heavy foods, however, given the wealth and luxurious habits of his patients, a difficulty compounded by their general inactivity and sedentary occupations – a problem familiar today. It is likely that Cheyne had read Cornaro and, paraphrasing the Venetian, he agreed with the idea that:

> since our wealth has increased and our navigation has been extended, we have ransacked all the parts of the globe to bring together its whole stock of materials for riot [and] luxury. The tables of the rich and great (and indeed of all ranks who can afford it) are furnished with provisions of delicacy, number and plenty, sufficient to provoke, and even gauge the most large and voluptuous appetites ... The whole controversy among us, seems to lie in outdoing one another in such kinds of perfusion.

Not only was the profusion of luxury foods newly available to wreck the health of the unwary, but a new perversion was threatening: 'a gross over-consumption of flesh and the degradation inherent in its production'. The meat that people were eating came from confined animals, 'physick'd almost out of their lives, and made as great epicures as those that feed on them'. The nervous diseases that plagued men were produced in the animals themselves (by their confinement and by treatments that included purging, bleeding and a feed of unnatural high-seasoned food) even before they were slaughtered and brought to the dinner table. The ways in which the meat was dressed and cooked was, Cheyne thought, 'carried on to an exaulted height, the ingenious mixing and compounding of sauces with foreign spices and provocatives, are contrived, not only to rouze a fickly appetite to receive the unnatural load, but to render a natural good one incapable of knowing when it has enough'.

Damning these carnivorous excesses, Cheyne told his patients that they alone had responsibility for their health, habits and self-discipline. This raised the idea that physicians were quite unnecessary rather than merely ineffectual (which they often were), and his medical peers were not best pleased. They retaliated, deriding the very idea that a 32-stone physician should be lecturing people on diet, and one Fellow of the Royal Society openly mocked him in his *Remarks on Dr Cheyne's Essay on Health and Long Life* (1724), saying that his advice 'may well please such as will flatter themselves, but can never save them from death'. Sneering at 'Dr Diet', he suggested that 'the Trick for making Men Immortal upon Asparagus and Parsnips' just wouldn't catch on. Another physician, 'Pillo-Tisanus', published an *Epistle to Ge——ge Ch——ne* in 1725:

O, Doctor, Doctor! – Who wou'd with you dine?
When your whole Bill of Fare is one starv'd Line,
Mutton six Ounces! – And a Pint of Wine!
… For my Physician I accept your Book;
But, by the Gods! – You ne'er shall be my Cook!

Cheyne was not to be moved and stuck to his maxim that a man is what he eats. He was evangelical in his zeal for vegetarianism, saying, 'I cannot find any great difference between feeding on human flesh and feeding on animal flesh, except custom and practice.' Vegetable recipe books were becoming more common, such as *Adam's Luxury* and *Eve's Cookery*, both available in the mid-1700s. Dr William Lambe (1765–1847) also advocated vegetarianism, associating it with cultivation, the arts, peace, agriculture and enlightenment, while meat-eating was aligned with inarticulate barbarianism. After some self-experimentation Cheyne came up with a light and low diet consisting mainly of milk and vegetables. This, he thought, was best combined with a programme of temperance and regular exercise and sleep. 'None ever failed or died,' he declared with confidence, 'who entered on a milk, seed, and vegetable diet.' This regimen also brought him the personal tranquillity and mental stability he longed for and, as if to vindicate his regimen, he lived into his early seventies despite his early life of reckless debauchery.

His friend Samuel Johnson (1709–84), however, got fatter and fatter as he got older. Johnson's *Dictionary of the English Language* defined diet as: 'food, provisions for the mouth; victuals', as well as 'food regulated by the rules of medicine, for the prevention and cure of any disease'. Sadly afflicted by his overweight body, Johnson was, like Cheyne, prone to melancholia, describing his depression as a black dog. Many physicians linked depression of the spirits to poor digestion and in particular to constipation, recommending soft diets and purging. Voltaire also had wise words to say on this problem: 'Persons who have an easy and regular movement every morning after they have breakfasted are the favourites of nature. They are sweet, affable, gracious, thoughtful, complaisant and efficient. A "no" in their mouths has more grace than a "yes" in the mouths of the constipated.'

Samuel Taylor Coleridge (1772–1834) was similarly concerned with bloating and constipation (unsurprisingly, given his predilection for opium). In his notebooks, on 13 May 1804, he described his 'Weight, Languor, & the soul-sickening Necessity of attending to barren bodily sensations, in bowels … the endless Flatulence, the frightful constipation when the dead Filth impales the lower Gut … to weep & sweat & moan & scream for the parturience of an excrement with such pangs & such convulsions as a woman with an Infant heir of Immortality'. The surgeon came immediately, he wrote, and then went back for his pipe and syringe and, with extreme difficulty and 'the exertion of his utmost strength injected the latter. Good God! – What a sensation when the obstruction suddenly shot up! – I remained still three-quarters of an hour with hot water in a bottle to my belly (for I was desired to retain it as long as I could) with pains & sore uneasiness, & indescribable desires – at length went. O what a time …' (Dorothy Wordsworth, in fact, expressively used the phrase 'bad bowels' in her journals as something of a pseudonym for Coleridge.)

An anonymous physician, writing an advice pamphlet on diet and regimen in the early nineteenth century, pitied the poor stomach and 'the violence which we offer it … the daily errors which we commit in the quantity and quality of our food'. The worst of all errors were the rich sauces and pastries. In fact, 'most confectionery must be placed in the forbidden list [and] the supper meal is obsolete,' he wrote. The state of one's digestive system and the excessive fat of many were not his only worries in the question of regimen: 'In proportion as luxury renders man effeminate, it requires from him nicer rules of management in diet.' In eighteenth-century America, meanwhile, cookbooks had twice as many pages on suet pies, pastries, cakes, custards, puddings and preserves as did the English equivalents. Visiting foreigners, 'Frenchmen, Germans, and even Englishmen, exclaim against our copious and everlasting dinners'. William Cobbett, an Englishman who visited America, wrote, 'You are not much asked, not much pressed, to eat and drink; but such an abundance is spread before you, and so hearty and so cordial is your reception, that you instantly lose all restraint, and are tempted to feast whether you be hungry or not', and 'though the manner and style are widely different in different houses, the abundance every where prevails'. One Charles Caldwell, a professor, remarked that, 'for every reeling drunkard that disgraces our country [America], it contains one hundred gluttons'.

Johnson believed that 'whatever be the quantity that a man

eats, it is plain that if he is too fat, he has eaten more than he should have done', and he did try to diet, recording in September 1780 that he had been 'attentive to my diet and have diminished the bulk of my body'. Johnson's biographer James Boswell, who as *The London Magazine*'s resident 'Hypochondriack' had a slightly broader view of the unfairness of the dieter's life, noted that 'you will see one man fat who eats moderately, and another lean who eats a great deal'. How could this be?

The idea that becoming overweight was simply a result of eating too much in relation to the energy expended was not the only view. Dr Thomas Beddoes (1760–1808) came up with a radical alternative theory on the causes of excess fat and the remedy of self-starvation. In 1793 he applied 'pneumatic chemistry' to the problem. This theory derived from M. Lavoisier's experiments in France which suggested that during respiration the lungs took in oxygen, combined it with carbon from food, and expelled it as carbon dioxide. Beddoes believed that oxygen might travel further into the body and that if it did not properly combine with body fat then it would accumulate rather than be burned up as energy (a defect of metabolism, in effect). He tried to remedy this by introducing more oxygen, but to no discernible good. 'No process in human life,' wrote Beddoes, 'is more common than sinning against the stomach and repenting shortly afterwards ... Compare what is lost and gained by throwing into the stomach materials that puff it up like a balloon.' Beddoes' contemporary, Dr William Wadd (1776–1829), rather unkindly rubbished his idea by remarking that, 'Dr Beddoes remained so inconveniently fat during this life that a lady of Clifton [in Bristol, where he lived and experimented] used to denominate him the walking feather bed'.

Wadd, Surgeon Extraordinary to the King and physician to the wealthy, was nonetheless appalled that polysarcia was so common that it existed 'without being deemed worthy of attention'. He became something of a celebrity for his *Cursory Remarks on Corpulence or Obesity Considered as a Disease* (1810), a publication that went to four editions during his lifetime, and in which he provided a graphic observation of a post-mortem examination of a very fat person: 'The heart itself was a mass of fat. The omentum was a thick fat apron. The whole of the intestinal canal was embedded in fat, as if melted tallow had been poured into the cavity of the abdomen … So great was the mechanical obstruction to the functions of an organ essential to life, that the wonder is, not that he should die, but that he should live.' In pursuit of a cure he looked at all the dieting advice he could find. The book's final section, a critical examination of ancient and modern opinions on excess fat, is an illuminating trawl through the favourite regimens of the time. Wadd especially recommended: eating bread chiefly made with bran, vegetables of all kinds, and only small quantities of meat; drinking little; eating salted meat; omitting tea and laying off the alcohol (he, along with other doctors, believed there was a danger of spontaneous combustion when alcohol was mixed with fat); taking very little sleep; applying a bandage to the abdomen and then tightening and relaxing it 'at pleasure'; taking digitalis; horseback riding; taking a sea voyage; reading aloud; walking more quickly than was usual; sprinkling the body with hot sand; sweating through the use of stoves and hot baths (as well as the occasional cold bath to strengthen and invigorate); bathing in medicated waters; sprinkling the body with salt; and strictly no vomiting after supper.

Wadd's thorough research also revealed the degrees to which physicians differed in their advice. The seventeenth-century physiologist Giovanni Borelli, Wadd found, advised chewing tobacco, others suggested vinegar of squills (a diuretic made from the bulb of an onion-like plant), abstinence and exercise, more oxygen in the system, plenty of fennel water, and a strict vegetable diet which 'reduces exuberant fat more certainly than any other means I know'. Vapour baths and shampooing were also recommended, and eating a bar of soap on a nightly basis was popular, either as an emetic or a laxative or, most likely, both. One patient of 20 stone took, each night for two years, 'at bedtime, a quarter of an ounce of common home-made castile soap dissolved in a quarter of a pint of soft water'. Another, a country gentleman, purchased 'a quarter of a hundredweight of castile soap, for the sole purpose of eating'. But purgatives, thought Wadd, were dangerous if used excessively and perspiration was pointless, so it was abstinence that won the day.

Having boiled down all the advice to three principal elements – diet, exercise and sleep – Wadd finally recommended a regimen devised by a Dr Schliecher, known as the 'little and often' diet. This is it:

7 a.m. Mutton or veal cutlet, or small sole, bread.
8 a.m. Cup of tea, with sugar.
10.30 a.m. Meat sandwich.
Noon. Meat, eggs, green vegetables, cheese, fresh fruit, a
    glass of white wine.
4 p.m. Cup of tea, with sugar.
7 p.m. Bread and cheese.
9 p.m. Cold meat, salad, and two glasses of white wine.

By the time of Wadd's own death in 1829, falling from a runaway carriage in Ireland, it was clear that being too fat was a commonplace complaint, that dieting was set to become a popular concern in the Victorian era, and that a new cultural aesthetic, with differing approaches to the politics and ethics of eating, was on the point of emerging. Luxury and excess in the face of others' starvation had brought revolution to France. In Britain in the 1790s and 1800s there were several crop failures, heavy taxation, and a hungry labouring class which was very aware of the extreme gluttony and decadence of the Prince of

Wales (later to be George IV). *The New Brighton Guide* of 1796 called his Brighton Pavilion a site of architectural waste and excessive oral consumption in which the prince and his hangers-on 'swill'd and reswill'd, and repeated their boozings, Till their shirts became dy'd with purpureal oozings'. Another said that this was why the 'nation at this day presents a picture of luxury, selfishness and general depravity, that was never equalled in the most abandoned age of Charles II'. Gillray's cartoons depicted George as supremely wasteful, parasitically feeding off the country: in a 'A Voluptuary under the Horrors of Digestion', he depicted the prince as a horribly bloated figure with a massively swollen stomach and obese thighs as he gourmandises among food debris and an overflowing chamber pot, a picture of filth and over-consumption. Fat here is stigmatised and associated with filth, greed and laziness.

The tyranny of gluttony had vexed the nineteenth-century consumer from the start. Food was an 'ensemble of beliefs, texts, practices and materials', and it raised 'questions about aesthetics and economics, the natural and the cultural, the social, the psychic and the biological'. There was a sense in which diet was sexualised, in that some foods, such as plain meat and vegetables, were appropriate to manly (that is 'good') behaviours, while others, such as spicy and sweet concoctions, were weak and effeminate, and all of it involved ecstasy and denial. Mary Wollstonecraft, in her *Vindication of the Rights of Women* (1792), wrote that, 'a very considerable number [of women] are, literally speaking, standing dishes to which every glutton may have access'. The preoccupation with weight began at birth. Jonathan Swift's *Modest Proposal* (1729) 'reckoned upon a medium that a child just born will weigh twelve pounds' – this was the opinion of the medical authorities of the time, and a quite arbitrary figure. In 1860, the Reverend David Macrae remarked that, 'One of the first things to be done with a baby when it is born, seems to be to hurry it into a pair of scales ... It continues to be weighed at short intervals all through its childhood, and on to the time when the question becomes one of personal interest and it is old enough to weigh itself.' The physiologist John Hunter (1728–93), Surgeon-General to George III, believed that the impetus of life lay in digestion rather than conception, and that digestion perpetuated life. The stomach was the chief organ of the human body, 'The converter of food by hidden powers into part of ourselves, and is what may be called the true animal, no animal being without it; and in many, perhaps in most, it is what constitutes the principal part of an animal.' His *Lectures on the Principles of Surgery* thus promoted healthy bodily functions as behavioural norms that brought stability – to the body and the body politic. A bloated state, of either kind, was a disaster.

These interconnecting ideas on diet, nature and political ethics excited influential figures such as Percy Bysshe Shelley (1792–1822) who campaigned for vegetarianism and published *A Vindication of Natural Diet* in 1813. Shelley, it has been said, was an enemy of sensuality with the diet of a hermit who sometimes couldn't have said if he had dined or not. This was ethical eating: it fitted with the recommendations of medicine, fed into the idea of temperance and self-control and was socially and politically responsible. It represented a return to 'nature', a contemporary reaction to pollution, artificiality and corruption that has resonance today. Shelley's *Swellfoot the Tyrant* (1820) concerns the political sufferings within the class system and depicts a grisly temple of famine that includes, among other decorations, a 'number of exceedingly fat Priests in black garments arrayed on each side with marrow-bones and cleavers in their hands'. Swellfoot is shown to be an exemplar of the swaggering, incontinent and corpulent villain, praising:

Kings and laurelled Emperors,
Radical-butchers, Paper-money-millers,

Bishops and deacons, and the entire army
Of those fat martyrs to the persecution
Of stifling turtle-soup, and brandy-devils ...

Shelley argued that the body was constructed, produced and consumed in society; he drew a straight line between lobster-boiling and Christian state despotism. The message was that diet, and therefore size, was political.

The distinguished naval medic Dr Thomas Trotter (1760–1832), a near contemporary of Shelley's, was similarly concerned with modern excess and contrasted it with an ancient, noble naturalness. In his view, the wealth, luxury, indolence and intemperance of town life was a 'vortex of dissipation', and the consumption of highly seasoned delicacies only hastened people's degeneration and the sinking of their souls in a 'gross body'. The epigraph to Trotter's *A View of the Nervous Temperament* (1807), which advocated a temperate diet, is a quotation from Macbeth:

Boundless intemperance
In Nature is a tyranny: it hath been
The untimely emptying of the happy throne,
And fall of many kings.

Mad, bad and dangerous to know, the notorious and charismatic Lord Byron (1788–1824) also happened to be a little fat. The embodiment of the Romantic poetic male – pale, thin and consumptive in his depictions – Byron actually had a 'morbid propensity to fatten'. Like celebrities today, Byron worked hard at maintaining his figure. When he went up to the University of Cambridge he began a strict diet regimen, both to get thin and to keep his mind clear, and this involved wearing layers of clothes to induce sweating. Acquaintances record his horror of fat, which he believed lead to lethargy, dullness and stupidity, and his anxiety that his creativity would be lost if he allowed himself to eat too much – or even normally. Byron starved and measured himself constantly and then, when quite famished, he binged, devouring huge meals that would be finished off with an overdose of magnesia to settle the stomach. He was both greedy and fastidious, a difficult combination. In his early thirties, while travelling in Italy, he kept mainly to a diet of claret and soda water but recorded in his Ravenna Journal on Friday, 26 January 1821, that 'On dismounting, found Lieutenant E. just arrived from Faenza. Invited him to dine with me to-morrow. Did not invite him for to-day, because there was a small turbot, (Friday, fast regularly and religiously,) which I wanted to eat all myself. Ate it.' His favourite slimming meal was biscuits and soda, and he once refused a voluptuous dinner, sticking to a new fad diet of potatoes flattened and drenched in vinegar.

Such was Byron's tremendous cultural power that the medical profession and the public worried about his malign influence on impressionable youth, in much the same way that fears are expressed today when footballers or libertine pop stars behave in a destructive and excessive way. Byron was accused of encouraging melancholia and emotional volatility – 'the dread of being fat weigh[ed] like an incubus' on Romantic youth who drank vinegar to lose weight and ate rice to give themselves a pale complexion – and of making girls sicken and waste away. If plump, they berated themselves as criminals against refinement and aesthetic taste, and prayed for a spell of illness to pull them down. The American physician, George Miller Beard (1839–83), who defined and named the condition of neurasthenia later in the century, fretted that young ladies lived all their growing girl-hood in semi-starvation because of their fears of 'incurring the horror of disciples of Lord Byron'. Beard made a direct association between the very popular Romantic movement and scanty eating, a slim body and delicacy of mind. According to Byron, 'a woman should never be seen eating or drinking, unless it be lobster salad and champagne, the only truly feminine and becoming viands' (actually, that doesn't sound too bad). But Byron's wit was underscored by cruelty and the double standard. When he ended his widely known and shocking affair with the married Lady Caroline Lamb, she lost so much weight through grief that Byron wickedly remarked to her mother-in-law that he was 'haunted by a skeleton'. By 1822 Byron had starved himself into an unnatural illness. Yet he was well aware of the effects of over-dieting, 'the cause of more than half our maladies'.

A letter that referred to Byron during a stay at the Villa Diodati in Switzerland in 1816, was quoted in *The Physiology of Taste or Meditations on Transcendental Gastronomy* (1825), by Jean-Anthelme Brillat-Savarin. The poet was dieting, it recorded, taking just 'a thin slice of bread with tea, at breakfast, a light vegetable dinner, with a bottle or two of seltzer water, tinged with Vin de Grave, and in the evening a cup of green tea without milk or sugar, [and this] formed the whole of his sustenance; the pangs of hunger he appeased by privately chewing tobacco and smoking cigars', tobacco being another well-known appetite suppressant.

Brillat-Savarin (1755–1826), a French lawyer, politician, lay physician and gourmet, was a very early proponent of the low-carbohydrate diet. Having escaped the Reign of Terror by moving to Switzerland and later New York, he returned to legal practice in France in 1797 and to the two great questions that faced the nation: Corpulency and Leanness. The destiny of a nation, he believed, following classical precepts, depended on how it nourished itself. So he wrote a diet book on the art of eating, on gastronomy, gourmandising, and the folly of '*recherché* dinners', *The Physiology of Taste or Meditations on Transcendental Gastronomy* (1825). This was a magisterial work with scientific pretensions. 'Everyone,' he confidently asserted, 'is desirous of avoiding corpulency, or of getting rid of it if, unhappily, he should have acquired it', and there was just one infallible method, founded upon the strict rules of physic and of science:

THAT A MORE OR LESS STRICT ABSTINENCE FROM ALL FARINACEOUS FOOD WILL TEND TO DIMINISH CORPULENCE.

Brillat-Savarin's 'anti-fat diet' was based on giving up the foods that he considered the 'commonest and most active cause of obesity': starches, sugars and farinaceous (flour-based) carbohydrate foods. These were the culprits, causing fatty congestion in people and animals, something amply demonstrated by the fattening of beasts for the markets. It was obvious that a more or less rigid abstinence from everything starchy or floury would lead to weight loss, especially if sugar went too. Instead, one should eat green and root vegetables, fruit and light meat, and drink water, coffee, tea, light white wines, and just the occasional spirit. 'Tell me what you eat,' he wrote, and 'I will tell you what you are' – a good and sensible start, before his comments descend into the casual misogyny of the period with, 'A dinner without cheese is like a pretty woman with only one eye.'

Although Brillat-Savarin believed that it was carbohydrates that made you fat, he continued to believe in the contemporary notion that self-starvation, too, was beneficial. Starvation, low-carbohydrate foods and exercise on foot or on horseback were his three absolute precepts. He himself had suffered from a fat belly ('seldom found in women') yet, he coquettishly remarked, he had 'an ankle, instep and calf, as firm as an Arabian horse'. His stomach, however, he regarded as a most formidable enemy and, after thirty years' effort, had conquered and reduced it to what he considered its proper dimensions. Hard work and dedication were involved ('grave efforts are rare exceptions'), but it was best if you only asked people to do what they found easiest to manage. It required, he knew from experience, 'great strength of character for a man to get up from the table while he is still hungry; as long as appetite lasts, one mouthful leads to another with irresistible attraction … in defiance of doctors and sometimes in imitation of them'.

Brillat-Savarin knew that people would think him a monster for depriving them of their favourite foods when all they had to do was avoid refined foods, fat, biscuits and such like, but: '"Oh Heavens!" all you readers of both sexes will cry out, "Oh Heavens above! But what a wretch the Professor is! Here in a single word he forbids us everything we most love, those little white rolls from Limet, and Achard's cakes, and those cookies … and a hundred other things made with flour and butter, with flour and sugar, with flour and sugar and eggs! He doesn't even leave us potatoes, or macaroni! Who would have thought this of a lover of good food who seemed so pleasant?"' But the alternative, he reminded them, was to get fat and 'become ugly, and thick, and asthmatic, and finally die in your own melted grease: I shall be there to watch it'.

For breakfast, dieters could have rye bread (less nourishing and, most importantly, less pleasant – but they could eat only the crust), absolutely no eggs, and drink chocolate rather than coffee. Breakfast was best had as early as possible so that one's digestion could complete itself before the next meal. Lovers of soup were allowed it à la julienne, with green and root vegetables, and cabbages. They had to leave off rice, breads, starchy pastes, flour and the crusts of hot pasties, but they could eat plenty of radishes, artichokes, asparagus, celery, cardoons, veal and poultry. Sugary dishes were forbidden, but they could choose a chocolate custard, jellies made with wine and orange juice, or fruit, fresh or preserved. After dinner they could have coffee, white wine or perhaps a liqueur, but should 'shun beer as if the plague'. If they were already fat then thirty bottles of seltzer water were to be drunk over a summer, two tumblers each morning before breakfast and before bed at night. If one wore Brillat-Savarin's patented restrictive Anti-Corpulency Belt, night and day, and gradually tightened it, it would keep the spine straight and stop the 'curving over which stretches the skin of the stomach so that it can't be retracted when weight is lost'. On top of all this dieters were exhorted to flee temptation and to remember that it was a question of morale. It was imperative, Brillat-Savarin believed, that the dieter developed a philosophical attitude to their predicament – an early nod at the importance of the psychology of dieting.

Brillat-Savarin was unwilling to label excess fat a disease: 'CORPULENCY IS NOT A MALADY; IT IS AT MOST A LAMENTABLE RESULT OF AN INCLINATION TO WHICH WE GIVE WAY, AND WE ALONE ARE TO BLAME.' But if it was plain to him that obesity was not actually a disease, it was without doubt 'a most unpleasant state of ill-health, and one into which we almost always fall because of our own fault'. It took willpower and determination to lose weight, and his diets were designed to help by matching a regimen to the temperament of the overweight individual. They were 'founded on the most solid precepts of both physics and chemistry [a] diet adapted to whatever effect is desired'. Of all possible medical prescriptions, the diet was the most important because it worked on the whole body, twenty-four hours a day. But drugs could help, too. Quinine had, he asserted, an anti-corpulent quality that disturbed fluids which might otherwise turn to fatty matter. He had observed people with fevers being treated with household remedies and with quinine, and those who had taken quinine had stayed thin. This, he deduced, was due to its stimulating effect. So, after the first month of a sensible diet, anyone who wished to grow thinner would do well, he argued, to take for the following month, every other day at seven in the morning, a glass of dry white wine in which has been dissolved about a teaspoonful of good red quinine, and that excellent results would soon follow.

He tried a new tack, thinking that an emphasis on the physical inconveniences of being fat might be more useful than moralising, more persuasive than sermons, and more powerful than laws, and that women would be more susceptible to this argument. Something had to persuade people that the pleasures of the table would finish them off: 'We, who believe ourselves to be the finest flower of civilisation, eat too much,' he warned, and 'enormous masses of foodstuffs and potables are absorbed every day without need'. An overweight Monsieur Louis Greffulhe came to Brillat-Savarin for help and was immediately made to promise that he would dutifully follow a diet and, as an article of faith, would weigh himself at the beginning and end of the treatment so that there might be a mathematical basis on which to judge the results. After one month Greffulhe reported that he had stuck to the rules as if his life depended on it and that he had lost at least three pounds. Not a huge amount, then, but he felt his sacrifices had been huge and he was giving up. The inevitable occurred, according to Brillat-Savarin. Greffuhle piled on the pounds and, although he was barely forty years old, died from breathing difficulties due to his weight. Gluttony and lack of willpower were his downfall; it took courage to lose weight and keep it off.

As for beauty, Brillat-Savarin, who regarded himself as an admirer of the finer things in life, wrote that 'corpulency has a baneful influence upon both sexes, inasmuch as it is detrimental to strength and beauty'. Excess fat, he wrote, made once-interesting faces almost insignificant, and nine out of ten 'corpulents' had round faces, globular eyes and pug noses. Napoleon I, for example, put on a lot of weight during his last campaigns and became pasty and dull. Musing on what he would have achieved had he been a physician, Brillat-Savarin thought he would first have written a detailed monograph on being fat, then would have established himself as an expert to 'enjoy the double advantage of having the healthiest of all patients on my list, and of being besieged daily by the prettier half of the human race, for it is the life study of all women to maintain a perfect weight, neither too heavy nor too light'. If a doctor treating overweight women was well-educated, discreet and good-looking, then Brillat-Savarin predicted miracles for him; and indeed many modern diet gurus fit this bill.

Women's 'primitive form and beauty' easily became buried beneath flesh, he thought, and when he met a 'charming little girl, with rosy cheeks and rounded arms, dimpled hands and a *nez retroussé*, and pretty little feet', Brillat-Savarin would look forward ten years and imagine her older and fatter. Fat made dancing, walking and riding more difficult and predisposed its 'victims' to illnesses such as apoplexy, dropsy, and ulcers on the legs, and it made everything harder to cure. But, still, it seemed, 'to tell a person of embonpoint to get up early in the morning, is to break his (or her) heart'. And riding didn't, he acknowledged, suit every-one; it was expensive and a woman would only do it if she had a handsome, lively and gentle horse, if she had a new riding habit tailored in the latest style, and if her groom was good-looking. Walking could be a nuisance, too, and hopelessly boring, appar-ently, as 'it is so fatiguing, the mud and the dust are dreadful, and the stones cut the pretty little boots, and then if a pimple the size of a pin's head should break out, it is immediately put down to that horrid doctor and his system, which is, of course, abandoned'.

If excess fat stole away a woman's beauty, then excess skinni-ness was no more preferable. According to Brillat-Savarin it was a 'horrible calamity for women: beauty to them is more than life itself, and it consists above all of the roundness of their forms and the graceful curvings of their outlines. The most artful toi-lette, the most inspired dressmaker, cannot disguise certain lacks, nor hide certain angles; and it is a common saying that a scrawny woman, no matter how pretty she may look, loses something of her charm with every fastening she undoes.' He wanted thin women to regain some of their plump flesh and to get rid of the silk and cotton padding which was commonly displayed in novelty shops, 'to the obvious horror of the prudish who pass them by with a shudder, turning away from such shadows with even more care than if it were the actuality they looked upon'. In order to put on fat, he recommended eating plenty of bread, baked fresh each day. Before 8 o'clock in the morning a thin woman should have a bowl of soup thickened with bread or noodles, and a cup of good chocolate. At 11 o'clock she must lunch on fresh eggs, scrambled or fried, a little meat pie or chops, and a cup of coffee. After lunch a little exercise wouldn't go amiss, a walk 'perhaps to the Tuileries, their dressmakers, the shops and to their friends'. At dinner she could have soup, meat and fish, rice and macaroni, frosted pastries, sweet custards and creamy puddings and, for dessert, Savoy biscuits and the popular contemporary pastry baba. She could have beer or wines from Bordeaux or the French Midi, even though all acids, especially vinegar, might lead to an early grave.

Brillat-Savarin told the tragic tale of a young lady friend whom he knew in Dijon in 1776, when he was studying law, chemistry and medicine:

> Louise —— was a lovely girl, and had the classical embon-point which charms the eye, and is the glory of sculptors. Though only a friend, I was not blind to her attractions, and this is perhaps why I observed her so closely. 'Chère amie,' I said to her one evening, 'you are not well; you seem to be thinner.' 'Oh! no,' she said, with a smile which partook of melancholy, 'I am very well; if I am a little thinner I can very well afford it.' 'Afford it!' I said, with warmth, 'you can afford neither to gain nor lose; remain beautiful as you are,' and other phrases pardonable to a young man of twenty. Since that conversation I watched her more closely, with an inter-est not untinged with anxiety; gradually I saw her cheeks fall

in, her figure decline. One evening at a ball, after dancing a quadrille, I cross-questioned her, and she reluctantly avowed that her school friends having laughed at her, and told her that in two years' time she would be as fat as St Christopher, she had for more than a month drunk a glass of vinegar every morning; she added that she not told anybody of it.

I shuddered when I heard her confession; I was aware of the danger she incurred, and next day I informed her mother, who was terribly alarmed, for she doted upon her child. No time was lost. The very best advice was taken. All in vain! The springs of life had been attacked at the source; and when the danger was suspected, all hope was already gone. Thus, for having followed an ignorant advice, poor Louise was carried to her grave in her eighteenth year, her last days embittered by the thought that she herself, involuntarily, had cut short her existence. She was the first person I ever saw die; she died in my arms, as, at her wish, I was raising her up that she might behold the light.

Brillat-Savarin did have a serious message about succumbing to obsessively self-imposed and dangerous regimens, diminished though it was by his fabulous self-aggrandising. Melodramatic and romantic, Brillat-Savarin's tragic tale deployed a shock effect in order to influence young women in much the same way that magazines and websites do today, although the motives of some of these are less noble, driven as they are by greed, profit and vested interests. Brillat-Savarin was one of a growing band of diet 'experts' who carved out a profitable niche for themselves in the early days of what would become the diet industry. With a credible theory, detailed dietary advice and celebrity anecdotes, Brillat-Savarin made use of a growing medical concern with polysarcia. He was in the vanguard of a new approach to diet that was reaching an increasingly large public audience, one with more money and more time to spend on itself.

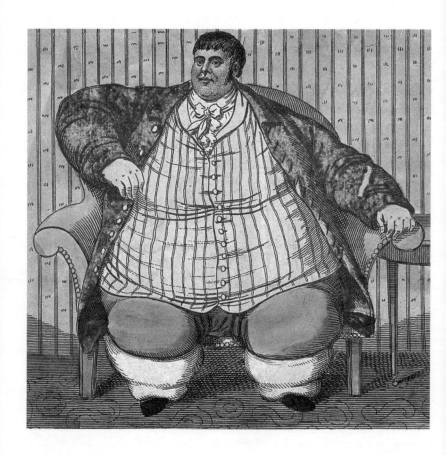

5. Very fat people have always attracted interest and ridicule. Daniel Lambert (1770–1809), above, was five feet, eleven inches tall as an adult and weighed fifty-two stones. He exploited his monstrous size as an entertaining curiosity for morbid onlookers, touring the country and charging for interviews. Today we have our newspapers, television and the internet to feed our need to gawp and to provide figures to measure ourselves against.

5

Advice to Stout People

EVERYONE WAS GETTING in on the diet act during the nineteenth century. Across Europe and America there were those, mostly men, who had set themselves up as experts and teachers, with diets to promote and products to sell. Sylvester Graham (1794–1851), inventor of the Graham Cracker, was an American Presbyterian minister whose dietary advice was coloured by his religious convictions. Gluttony, he railed, was easily the worst dietetic error in the United States, and probably the whole civilised world. Graham's regimen advised the elimination of meat, sauces, tea, coffee, alcohol, pepper and mustard, and advocated instead plenty of vegetables, whole-wheat bread, fruits, nuts and salt, and pure water to drink. He urged people to treat their stomach like a well-governed child: find out what was good for it and teach it to conform. The idea that the head should be governed by the stomach, instead of the other way round, he wrote, was wrong. Graham prescribed control of a different sort, a moral education that would become habit and, thereafter, 'what is commonly called nature'. The stomach, he wrote, should be 'the helpful minister of your body, and not the whole body the mere locomotive appendage of your stomach'.

A self-proclaimed 'Minister of the Interior' published his *Memoirs of a Stomach, Written by Himself, That All Who Eat May Read* (1853) in an attempt to lighten things up a little with satire. On his personal appearance he wrote, 'I must acknowledge, [it] is not prepossessing, as I resemble a Scottish bagpipe in form, the pipe being the oesophagus or gullet, and the bag myself. I often wish there were more "stops", especially when I am played upon by gluttony.' On the daily diet he suggested that at breakfast one should drink only black tea with very little sugar, and partake of a small French roll. Then, at noon, perhaps a light lunch of a small mutton chop or sandwich without butter, accompanied by a glass of ale, sherry or wine, 'as it is necessary to stave off excessive hunger till a late dinner'. 'Earn your dinner,' he cajoled, and leave the table as soon as you politely can, to join the ladies. And at night 'it is well to keep a little reserve of biscuit by the bed-side'. All stomachs, he continued, undoubtedly have their own peculiar idiosyncrasy and the 'especial points of my obstinacy may be summed up in a few general rules; and the first is MODERATION'. Secondly, 'if by any chance you should sacrifice to Epicurus a little too devotedly, all I ask is to give me REST'. A proper 'REGULARITY OF MEALS is another essential point' and, referring to the problems of constipation, he urged that 'EXERCISE, too, is a sine qua non, for the entire internal machinery becomes clogged unless a healthy waste of the system is produced by walking or riding'. Then there was 'MASTICATION, another highly important item in my economy … the next dietetic rule I desire you to observe is, NEVER TO DINE BY YOURSELF'. One should avoid when at all possible PHYSIC (medicines), too, and always follow a STRICT REGIMEN. The 'Minister' further advised rising tolerably early and performing one's ablutions all over with tepid water, rubbing oneself well dry, getting as red as a boiled lobster, and then follow this up by taking a brisk walk for half an hour. If the stomach should still inconveniently crave more food, then one could munch on a dry biscuit while going about one's daily business, rejoicing all the while. And possibly feeling a little smug.

This approach, which spoke so directly to the dieting individual, was also pursued by some enlightened members of the medical profession who recognised that the fat person needed support, motivation and organisation if their diet and change of regimen was to succeed. A member of the Royal College of Surgeons, Dr A. W. Moore, published a series of letters in the 1850s taken from the *Medical Times and Gazette*, which he called *Corpulency; I.e. Fat, or, Embonpoint, in Excess ... Explaining Briefly his Newly-Discovered DIET SYSTEM, to Reduce the Weight and Benefit the Health* (1856). That it ran to three editions in one year shows how popular it was. Moore's radical innovation was in giving over some thirty pages of his book to a 'Diet Diary'. This very modern innovation was laid out in columns and sections for the reader to complete, with spaces to be filled in with whatever he or she ate each day, and at what time, for Breakfast, Dinner, Tea and Supper. At the end of each day's record was a space for recording your weight. This was a ruthlessly organised system of watchfulness and intent. Moore included a synopsis of Cornaro's famous dieting story as a successful model for this way of eating and living.

A very favourable write-up of Moore's work in *The Morning Post* on 20 March 1857 attributed his successful 'little work' to the results of time, experience and thorough observation. The potential dieter who bought the book would not, it said, suffer disappointment, 'as without any further medical aid than the pamphlet affords, he can set to work to lessen the weight of his body. The plan of treatment is simple, and its explanation devoid of all medical mystification.' As well as providing a straightforward plan and framework for action, 'the author deserves to be ranked among those who have made a useful and scientific discovery'. Moore's medical training, based, as was then standard, on the precepts of classical medicine, as well as his own experience of cases, led him to prioritise the influence of the digestive system on the entire human constitution.

Nevertheless, Moore understood that promoting his diet plan could result in some negative publicity if the diet failed, as well it might – not because it wasn't effective, but because dieters were unreliable. Moore knew that sticking to a diet could be very hard work, full of temptations and pitfalls. Moreover, because medicine at this time was still a marketplace and a doctor's reputation and livelihood rested on his success rate, there was much rivalry, scepticism, and 'a good deal of unnecessarily morbid sensibility and irritability among us, scarcely found in any other liberal profession'. So, in the modern spirit of good publicity, he asked that the dieter not mention to anyone that he or she was on his plan 'until the effect is produced', that way neither he nor the dieter would be seen to fail and the potential customer would have proof of the diet's efficacy. Moore may also have felt exposed, as he recognised that it was 'impossible to gather any information respecting the cure of this ailment from the numerous authors who have written works on the practice of medicine' because the whole subject of dieting was so little understood. This uncertainty was simultaneously frustrating and to his advantage.

The way in which the general public would not hesitate to ridicule what 'appears in the person of another unavoidable, especially if it be some prominent feature', especially fat, was abhorrent to Moore. 'Much satire has been bestowed, even from olden times, upon the corpulent,' he wrote, 'some groaning at it, considering fat to be a curse in disguise; some pitying; while others go so far as to be enraged at it altogether, considering the possessors of an obese burden gourmands, monopolisers of the table, great sleepers, indolent, dull of comprehension, slow coaches.' Edward Bright, a grocer at Malden in Essex, was a famous 'figure of fun' in the mid-eighteenth century. At 5 ft 9 in. tall, he weighed 44 stone, and measured 5 ft 6 in. around the chest, 6 ft 1 in. around his waist; his arms were 2 ft 2 in. in circumference and each leg 2 ft 8 in. He was said to drink a gallon of small beer a day until he died at the age of thirty in 1750. After his death seven men were buttoned into his coat without stretching the seams, such was the astonishment his size engendered.

Bright had come from a family of fat people, unlike the famously huge Daniel Lambert, who was born in Leicester in 1770. Lambert was apparently quite 'normal' in appearance and appetite until his adolescence when he began to get fatter and fatter, despite his alleged plain diet. In 1806 Lambert was such a size that he travelled down to London in a specially constructed coach, and at 53 Piccadilly was charging a shilling a time for interviews. He was 5 ft 1 in. tall, 52 stone in weight, and he measured 3 ft 1 in. around each leg and 9 ft 4 in. around his torso. When he died, aged just thirty-nine, it was said that 'Nature had endured all the trespass she could admit. Corpulency constantly increased until the clogged machinery of life stood still, and this prodigy of Mammon was numbered with the dead.' Lambert's coffin, specially constructed, was built on wheels and was rolled through the streets to his grave. 'I believe no Age did ever afford more Instances of Corpulency than our own,' lamented an eighteenth-century physician, Thomas Short. The French Revolutionary and journalist Mirabeau once said of an excessively fat man that God had created him for the sole purpose of demonstrating the limits to which human skin could stretch without bursting.

In the 1880s, the *New York Daily Tribune* had reported on the people queuing up for the 'Two Tons of Fat on Exhibition' at Bunnell's Museum and for their chance to shake the fat men's flesh 'just to see it shiver'. There may have been a desire to enjoy the 'badness' of fat in the face of the medical profession's advice on how and what to eat. Even in 1937 it was reported that 'these curiosities and anomalies survive still for the amuse-ment of morbid onlookers at sideshows in fairs and circuses, but laughter at the expense of the unfortunate victims is now confined only to the obese, and even that is considered in these day as questionable taste'. Now such commentaries appear on the internet, on television or in the tabloid newspapers. And the shockingly thin have an audience, too, with their own websites. While the personal has always been political, the personal is also increasingly in the public eye. No wonder, then, that there is a growing problem with distorted body image worldwide, with catastrophic effects on mental and physical health.

Before he wrote *Corpulency*, Dr Moore had suffered ridicule himself, when a medical student and weighing some 15½ stone. He managed, with his diet system, to reduce in three months to 12½ stone by breakfasting early on two ounces of (an Abernethy or captain's) biscuit, one egg and two cups of tea or coffee. Then he fasted until five when he had a dinner consisting of 'animal food, etc.'. In particular, he took care to eat no bread at all.

Moore's diet plan consisted, then, of steady perseverance, good sleep (he thought it a fallacious idea that sleep could make you fat), avoiding bread and fermented liquor, and fasting between the hours of nine and five. He was adamant that people should do away with the notion that vinegar was an antidote to corpulency, a belief that was, in his opinion, as well as Brillat-Savarin's, 'apt to haunt the minds of young ladies who are desir-ous of becoming celebrated for an elegant slenderness of form'. He knew of one such young flibbertigibbet who diminished her food intake for a year, went horse-riding as severe exercise, and drank large quantities of vinegar each day with the result that she developed dyspepsia, hysteria, a dry cough, pungent pains in her side, hectic sweats, occasionally purulent expectoration and was pronounced to be in the last stages of consumption, her life posi-tively despaired of. All of this was only averted at the last moment by a physician who had the foresight to prescribe the gradual renewal of a nutritious diet and some fortifying tonics. Moore also thought vegetarianism was a pointless, antique notion. Out walking one day in the Strand in 1851, the year of the Great Exhibition, he had come across a sign for an enormous fat woman exhibiting herself and, on paying his money with a view to questioning her and the exhibitor, he was surprised to find that they were rigid vegetarians. Not only that but, astonishingly to him, 'she was not at all a little proud of belonging to that (doubtless erroneous) way of dieting'. Elaborate and excessive exercise was equally ineffective he thought, though he advised regular, moderate exertion, suggesting perhaps the odd game of quoits.

Moore himself was, in his own estimation, a 'constitutionally fat' man and, despite 'Corpulency, i.e. Fat' being a necessary ingredient of the body, nature was sometimes, unfortunately, too liberal in its supply. In men, even though 'a more than moderate supply of fat aids motion', it could be a terrible inconvenience. However, for women, who were not expected to be physically active, things were a little different because, in line with the beauty ideal of the time, 'in the female [fat] improves the beauty of the person'. To be very stout, however, was in his opinion no addition to beauty, although he warned that 'ladies particularly, while most anxious to find out the secret to becoming thin, often resort to means likely to affect their health, and produce a variety of unpleasant symptoms; this is an unwise and dangerous proceeding, for mere sake of personal appearance'.

Moore also had some curious notions about the causes of fat. He did not, for example, want to rule out the influence of the atmosphere which, he wrote with confidence, 'has sometimes the effect of producing a very great accumulation of fat'. To back up this vague assertion, which possibly had its roots in the miasmatic theory of disease – that sicknesses might arise from bad air – he asserted that, 'it has been observed that in the short space of twenty-four hours, a mist will occasionally fatten snipes, wood-cocks, partridges, and many other birds, to such a degree that they can hardly get out of the way of the sportsman's gun'. The possibility that birds fluff up their feathers against the chill and become lethargic appears not to divert him from this idea. He also posited that 'Rage and vexation will often diminish in a very short time the plump appearance of many insects, by causing a greater amount than usual of carbonic acid gas to be excreted through the lungs.' For instance, he wrote, 'take a good fat bumble bee, which has gained his embonpoint by living on the sugar extracted from different plants, place him in a thin cardboard box, and weigh him; it will be found that, being vexed with his confinement, and humming out his anger, the increased action of the lungs will soon cause to be decomposed the excess of carbon in the system, and thus very soon diminish his weight'.

The wilder speculative musings of the doctor did not, however, seriously undermine his reliance on medical observation and experience. Alongside the useful Diet Diary, Moore's book gave case histories of people who had come to him for help in losing weight. One 'EW', a magistrate, 6 ft 3 in. tall, fifty-eight years old and weighing 21 stone, was 'suffering from or enjoying the true obesity of Prince Hal's jovial companion, viz. *Polysarcia Omenti*'. (This was a troublesome protuberance of the abdomen, a pot belly, as opposed to *Polysarcia Generalis*, a general obesity diffused equally over the body and limbs). EW followed Moore's diet and, he reported, it did the trick splendidly. Another, a brewer, wrote to Moore to tell him: 'I am a tremendous big fellow, about six feet two inches in height, and too stout by a great deal. Just lay down the law with respect to my diet and I will endeavour to abide by it.'

A third case was that of a young lady described as dwarfish in stature and so 'exceedingly fat that her head appeared fairly buried in her shoulders'. She had consulted many doctors who all pronounced her case hopeless, agreeing that her heart was in a state of fatty degeneration. Moore set her on his diet system and a month later she was much 'altered and improved' but, 'in the usual manner of patients when they are getting better [she] became the victim of oblivion in respect of her medical adviser'. Then, two years later, he was called to her again only to discover that she had suffered an apoplectic fit, for 'considering herself well she had relapsed into her former habit of taking much bread, and heavy fermented liquors, such as porter, which caused her to regain her usual bulk'. She had lapsed badly, succumbed quickly, and 'rallied for a few days only'. Diligence and proper management were the keys to success, wrote Moore.

Despite his apparent faith in these virtues, Moore did consider the possibility of corpulency as a disease, and a hereditary one at that, 'endemic in some countries'. Though the average weight of the human body was generally, he wrote, 140 lb and 6 oz (about 10 stone or 63.5 kilos), he noted that Americans were proverbially lanky, the Irish and Scots had comparatively few fat persons, and both the French and Italians were mostly lean though they ate a great deal of bread. On this last problem he insisted that 'we must remember that their disposition is very excitable, and almost every word spoken by them is accompanied by some quick movement of the body [so] there must necessarily be a great demand for much carbon and hydrogen, the chemical constituents of fat, which is consumed by the actions of the lungs and liver, as well as by that of the muscles. Our gay neighbours when excited seem to quiver from head to foot.'

The 'construction of fat is very peculiar,' he thought, and looking under his microscope he saw a mystery 'made up of isolated cells which contain within them the power of getting fatty substance out of the blood'. These, he divined, clustered together and were 'surrounded by little envelopes made of tissue'. The liver in constitutionally thin people, he argued, was 'generally very strong and able to separate and throw off from the blood any superfluity of its fatty and carbonaceous constituents'. This went some way to answering the 'curious and interesting question ... why are not all mankind fat?' and why, also, some people were able to eat plentifully and yet appear lean. It was a genetic as well as a dietary problem.

In the 1850s the European medical profession was beginning to accept the theory that carbohydrate and fat supplied the carbon that combined with oxygen in the lungs to produce body heat. This was the work of a German chemist, Baron Justus von Liebig (1803–73), and he argued that excessive fat was an overindulgence in carbohydrate and fat, 'respiratory foods', and that the accumulation of body fat was reliant upon these two being 'digested in greater quantities than is necessary to supply carbon to the respiration'. So the main treatment for obesity was to stop the supply of these foods, particularly fat, with an 'hourly watch over the instinctive desires', by which was meant self-starvation.

One man on a mission to rescue people from 'rash experiments', Dr Watson Bradshaw, published *On Corpulence* (1864) to give the overweight a strategic programme. First, he devised one of those all-too familiar questionnaires to ascertain whether you really were, objectively, fat, and whether you needed to do anything about it. Dr Bradshaw's questions ran as follows:

Are you well?
Do you sleep well?
Do you feel drowsy after dinner?
Can you walk fast with comfort?
Does your heart beat rapidly and forcibly when you ascend
    stairs?
Does a little exertion tire you?
Do you snore at night?
Can you stoop comfortably to put on your boots?

Can you walk at the rate of four miles an hour for twenty
minutes, with comfort?
Can you perform all that is desirable for a person of your
years?

Answer these questions correctly, wrote Bradshaw, and you
avoid the many miseries of 'extraordinary self-denial'. For those
whom the questionnaire proved overweight there were increasing numbers of new diets on offer. Nowadays, everyone knows
someone who has been on the Atkins diet, a system hailed as
a 'revolution' by its author in the 1970s, yet one of the earliest
low-carbohydrate diets to reach a major audience was the fan-
tastically popular Banting System which appeared to be followed
religiously by absolutely everybody.

This diet, first published in 1863 as a *Letter on Corpulence,
Addressed to the Public* by William Banting, when he himself had
lost forty-six pounds in a year, soon became so well-known that
'Banting' – as in 'I am Banting' – became a synonym for dieting
in the UK and America well into the 1920s. It is still commonly
used in Sweden (where 'Nej, tack, jag bantar' translates as 'No
thank you, I am dieting'). The term is mentioned, for instance,
in H. L. Mencken's *The American Language* and it turns up in
popular novels of the time, including Agatha Christie's crime
thrillers. So much diet information was published from the mid-
Victorian period onwards that one anonymous physician had
even published a book called *How to Get Fat* (1865), grouchily
remarking that people everywhere were asking each other, 'Have
you read Banting?' and moaning that it had become quite 'the
bon mot of the day'.

Banting (1797–1878) was a London undertaker to the wealthy
and fashionable – he had built the Duke of Wellington's coffin –
who lived just a few doors down from the wine merchant Berry
Bros. & Rudd, in St James's. This establishment had embraced
the late eighteenth-century European vogue for weighing oneself

at shops on large hanging scales (bathroom scales are an early twentieth-century phenomenon), and the records at Berry Bros. & Rudd reveal that the Earl of Salisbury weighed 15 st 9 lb in 1787, and 19 st 4 lb in 1798; and that Lord Byron was 13 st 12 lb in 1806, but was down to just 9 st by 1811. The vain dandy, Beau Brummell, weighed himself at the shop more than forty times between 1815 and 1822. Having become fatter and fatter throughout his adult life, Banting had made repeated attempts to reclaim his figure: one recommendation to stick to 'light food' had, for instance, laid him physically and mentally low, so much so in fact that he had broken out in boils and two enormous carbuncles which had necessitated surgery. Although never what we might now consider huge, Banting's weight also caused him to be admitted to hospital twenty times in as many years; and the regimens which he tried included swimming, walking, riding, taking the sea air and the spa waters at Leamington, Cheltenham and Harrogate, and having Turkish baths at a rate of up to three a week for a year. He drank 'gallons of physic and liquor potasse' and tried low-calorie, starvation diets, but he managed to lose only six pounds in all that time while, moreover, finding that he had less and less energy. By 1862, when he was sixty-five, Banting weighed 202 lb (14 st 6 lb) at just 5 ft 5 in. tall and, he wrote, 'I could not stoop to tie my shoes, so to speak, nor attend to the little offices humanity requires without considerable pain and difficulty which only the corpulent can understand. I have been compelled to go downstairs slowly backward to save the jar of increased weight on the knee and ankle joints and have been obliged to puff and blow over every slight exertion, particularly that of going upstairs.'

In desperation Banting consulted a noted Fellow of the Royal College of Surgeons, Dr William Harvey. Harvey, an ear, nose and throat specialist, had recently returned from Paris where he had heard a physiologist, Dr Claude Bernard, discussing a new theory about the part the liver played in cases of diabetes.

Bernard said that the liver, as well as secreting bile, also produced a sugar-like substance that it made from elements of the blood passing through it – it was well-known that a saccharine and farinaceous diet was used to fatten some farm animals. Harvey began to consider the roles of the various food elements in diabetes and started research on how fats, sugars and starches affected the body. Banting presented the opportunity for experiment and so Harvey devised a diet for him which was so successful that by Christmas Banting was down to 184 pounds, and to 156 pounds by the following August.

Banting published the revolutionary diet book privately and at his own expense, thinking that the editor of the *Lancet,* where he first thought of presenting it, would not want to publish anything 'from an insignificant individual without some special introduction'. He was right. Despite giving all the credit to Dr Harvey he was roundly attacked as unscientific and ignorant. Critics at the time included Josiah Oldfield who published *Starch as a Food in Nature, Being a Reply to the Anti-Starch Crusade* and, later, Francis W. Crowninshield writing in *Vanity Fair* in 1908, quipped that 'Banting has almost done away with the ancient custom of eating, but thyroid tablets and lemon juice are, of course, permitted'.

When Banting's pamphlet sold worldwide, thousands of grateful people wrote to thank him for the diet and tell him of their own success. Some had been lost to 'the wilderness of obesity', others 'not ridiculously fat, but inconveniently so'. All had, however, rid themselves of many unwanted pounds. One of these stoical dieters wrote that she could not say that she liked Banting's diet, 'but that is of no consequence' – a sentiment echoed by the dieting millions ever since. Although those on Banting's diet were told not to eat less and, particularly, not to starve themselves, Dr S. Weir Mitchell, a contemporary American physician, reported treating a woman who, he said, had 'been made very ill owing to an attempt to reduce her flesh by too rapid Banting'. In his essay *Fat and Blood* Mitchell wrote up the case history of a Mrs P. who at forty-five years old weighed 190 lb, was 5 ft 4 in. tall, was obese and anaemic and 'had for some years been feeble, unable to walk without panting, or to move rapidly even a few steps'. He put her on an exclusive milk diet and she lost one pound a day for thirty days. After the third week they included a little broth into her regimen, plus lactate of iron, Swedish exercises and massage. By week seven Mrs P.'s weight had dropped to 145 lb, a loss of forty-five pounds.

At the start of the day Banting urged dieters to begin with a tablespoon of a special alkaline corrective cordial in a wine glass of water, then at breakfast:

> 5–6 oz beef mutton, kidneys, broiled fish, bacon or cold meat – NOT pork or veal
> A large cup of tea or coffee (without milk or sugar)
> A little biscuit, or 1 oz of dry toast (generally taken with a tablespoon of spirit to soften it)
> Total: 6 oz of solids, 9 oz of liquids

At Lunch:

> 5–6 oz of any fish, except salmon, herrings or eels. Any meat, but NOT pork or veal
> Any vegetable, except potatoes or root vegetables
> 1 oz of dry toast
> Unsweetened fruit out of a pudding (i.e. cooked)
> Any kind of poultry or game
> 2 or 3 glasses of good claret, sherry or madeira
> Total: 10–12 oz of solids, 10 oz of liquids

For Tea:

2–3 oz cooked fruit
1–2 rusks
A cup of tea (without milk or sugar)
Total: 2–4 oz of solids, 9 oz of liquids

At Dinner:

3–4 oz meat or fish, as at lunch
1–2 glasses of claret, or sherry and water
Total: 4 oz of solids, 7 oz of liquids

For a nightcap, if you needed one, you might have a tumbler of grog (gin, whisky, or brandy without sugar) or 1–2 glasses of claret or sherry.

The Banting System advocated what was, at heart, a long-term, protein-rich, high-fat, low-carbohydrate diet plan. Dieters were advised to eat differently: to scrupulously avoid milk, sugar, starches, beer and butter, and to leave off champagne, salmon, herrings, eels, pork, veal, potatoes, parsnips, beetroot, turnips, carrots, puddings, pastries and port.

As *Punch* magazine put it in 1869:

If you wish to grow thinner diminish your dinner,
And take to light claret instead of pale ale;
Look down with an utter contempt upon butter,
And never touch bread till it's toasted – not stale.

'I've done it,' said brave Mr Banting,
And so may each overfed Briton,
If he'd only adopt resolution severe
And avoid – if he would not grow fatter and fatter,
All bread, butter, sugar, milk, 'taters and beer.

Richard MacKarness, who wrote *Eat Fat and Grow Slim* in 1958, calculated that in terms of calories Banting's diet added up to the 'astonishing' figure of 2,800 when an 'average modern low-calorie reducing diet allows a meagre 1,000 calories a day'. There must therefore have been something other than calorie reduction responsible for Banting's weight loss. The diet consisted almost entirely of protein, fat, alcohol and roughage. He himself said that he could quite confidently confirm that 'QUANTITY of diet may be safely left to the natural appetite; and that it is the QUALITY only which is essential to abate and cure corpulence': it was the carbohydrate (starch and sugar) that fattened fat people.

The mode of life of an ordinary Englishman tended, according to Dr Nathaniel Davies, to 'foster an accumulation of fat which prevents him taking exercise' and as the 'individual becomes so entangled in its toils, he or she finds, when it becomes necessary to grapple with it the power to do so curtailed, and the effort of taking the necessary steps so burdensome as to be practically impossible or too painful to continue'. As the fat 'crept on so invidiously and slowly' the fat person needed help – and he was the man to do it, and do it he would with the aid of science. Davies's book, *Food for the Fat: A Treatise on Corpulency with Dietary for Its Cure* (1889), emphasised the need to consult a physician. For corpulency was, Davies believed, definitely a disease.

This tendency, to categorise excess fat as symptomatic of disease, became increasingly popular with the medical profession as the nineteenth century progressed, providing a ready market – the overweight would, by definition, be wealthy – for exploitation. Patients were, on the whole, an ignorant lot, and quite liable to purge and starve themselves for short periods, doing serious harm and making the remedy worse than the disease. Or they might consult some utter quack who would reduce their balance at the bank but not their 'corporeal redundancy'. Under these circumstances, concluded Davies, life became no less than a burden for them. It was the 'nervous influence', you see: while the highly strung were seldom obese, 'on the other hand, the stupid, heavy, non-intellectual person, or the idiot, is generally fat and flabby'. However, and here he hedges his bets, there were examples of 'considerable intellectual attainments ... amongst the corpulent'. The intelligent, or those who considered themselves to be so, would not want to be thought of as idiotic, stupid or heavy, and this humiliating possibility was Davies's spur to them to lose weight. First he sympathised with the fat and then he insulted them into dieting – an effective tactic still used today by those selling diet foods, drinks and drugs. Buy a copy of *Foods for the Fat*, Davies proposed, and you could learn how to diet back to health without losing the 'pleasures of the table'.

The 'fat disease' was exacerbated by excess of food, especially certain kinds of food, too little work and a sedentary lifestyle, as well as the demon drink. The way back to health was as follows:

1. To improve by exercise the muscular tissue, and by diet to keep the muscles of the body in firm fibre and tone.
2. To maintain the blood.
3. To regulate the quantity of fluid in the body.
4. To prevent the deposit of fat, by eliminating from the diet an excess of those articles which create it, but are not otherwise useful in economy.
5. To allow quite sufficient food, and even many luxuries, so as to satisfy the cravings of nature and the wants of the system, and to do this in a gradual, harmless manner.

These instructions boil down to the same fundamental causes and remedies that would have been familiar to the Greeks and to most of the diet advisers that succeeded them. Care of the digestive system was paramount in avoiding disease brought on by being fat. Dr Edward Blake followed this classical argument in *Constipation and Some Associated Disorders* (1900). The wise would pay no attention to charlatans who promised to cure corpulency without a change of habit or diet, he wrote, but even 'physicians have devised the most extraordinary methods for reducing fat, by which possibly some thousands have been cured to death'. The absurdity of these cures consisted in trying to substitute one abnormality for another, by endeavouring to compensate for insufficient muscular work by insufficient nourishment. If a 'plump person be replacing muscular by adipose tissue ... such an one is not a proper man – he is corpulent', and the 'history of such people is that often they only leave the easy chair, to roll into bed!'

Next to water the most important element in food was fat, Blake maintained, and to suddenly give it up was nothing short of exceedingly perilous. And by fat he meant any oily food at all. Blake argued, somewhat against the grain, that it was quite wrong to think that fat people had just overdone the carbohydrates: 'OBESITY IS IN ALL CASES DUE TO INSUFFICIENT EMPLOYMENT OF THE MUSCLES. A person taking bodily exercise doesn't become fat, whatever form of diet he adopts.' Abdominal massages could be given three times a day before meals, to help with digestion and constipation, but such treatments could go too far. The massage technique practised at the popular Baden-Baden spa was particularly vigorous: the 'physician sinks his two fists as deeply as possible into the abdomen of the patient', then pinching, 'he grasps between the palms of his hands large pieces of the abdominal walls and squeezes them as forcibly as possible, in such a way as to crush the subcutaneous fat lobules. The force employed is so great that the patient's skin is covered with bruises. This is a most painful kind of massage and often extracts groans and tears from the patient!' The doctor then kneels on the abdomen and this,

Blake remarks, is torture and the brutality is surprising as 'fat people have indeed a deceptive appearance of vigour, whereas in reality, they are less robust than lean people'. They are obliged to undergo hot baths, too, lasting twenty minutes, with parts of the body bathed in different shaped baths, never the whole body at once. The initial temperature was set at 99.5 degrees Fahrenheit, progressively rising to 122 degrees. These were 'extremely painful' and Blake thought the cure seemed much worse than the disease and he knew that the English patients who flocked to Germany to be pummelled 'certainly would not tolerate such treatment in their own country'.

Extraordinary and wild theories on diets, on what exactly fat was and what could be done about an excess of it, were becoming increasingly, perhaps madly, popular in this period, and sometimes there was no mincing of words or fear of offending delicate sensibilities. Many diet books and pamphlets were one-off, fanatical, self-confessional works and ranged from the no-nonsense hard-hitting to the philosophical. There was one to cater for every class or cultural or political leaning. *The Cloven Hoof: An Epic for Epicures, and a Philosophical Text Book Containing the Secret of Long Life* (1895) by A. M. S. Roskruge was advertised as 'The Most Eccentric Book Ever Published' and contained some terrible poetry, gothic illustrations, quotes and aphorisms. The anonymous author of *Advice to Stout People: Showing How I Reduced from 20 Stone to 13 Stone with Full Particulars as to Diet, Treatment, Etc.* (1883), might have wanted to protect his identity but had reason other than embarrassment about his size for doing so. He, D— S— , had also published *Where to Dine and Where Not to Borrow: From Practical Experience*, and *Prison Life: Eighteen Months' Imprisonment (with a Remission)*.

A familiarity with the harsh Victorian prison system and a satirical sense of the absurdities of life gave D— S— a unique take on what to do about obesity. He would, he said, 'in fact make obesity penal, so calling for special legislation, whereby the police would be justified in arresting the oleaginous pedestrians, slapping them into the scales at the nearest police station, and if they exceed a certain number of feet in circumference or weight, at once procure their summary imprisonment, without the option of a fine. The streets would thus be cleared of the fleshy obstructions; besides which, if the Law recognises attempted suicide as a crime in one way, why not in another?' Shock tactics taken care of, he turned to diet as a remedy, specifically one which reflected the prison diet he had endured while incarcerated at Her Majesty's Pleasure, and limited to no more than two pounds of solid food and three pints of fluid per day:

6 a.m. – half pt black coffee, 1 oz coarse brown bread or biscuit.

9 a.m. – 4 oz lean meat, 3oz coarse brown bread or biscuit, and half pt black coffee.

2 p.m. – 6 oz lean meat, 3 oz coarse brown bread or biscuit, 6 oz green vegetables, and half pt fluid, not beer or effervescent wine or water.

After Dinner – half pt black coffee.

6 p.m. – half pt black coffee.

At Supper – 2 oz coarse brown bread or biscuit, and a couple of glasses of sherry or claret.

Fruit *ad lib*.

Liquorice powder, one teaspoon in water at bedtime.

There's an astonishing amount of coffee in this appalling diet – two pints a day – so he must have been very tense though coffee can, of course, be a diuretic and a purgative as well as a stimulant. In contrast, vegetables don't figure very much as he regarded them, especially root vegetables, as the 'fat person's poison', though for no obvious reason. The main thing was that he deemed it 'absolutely imperative to limit the quantity as well as the quality' of foods, thus possibly ruining the appetite in a two-pronged action. He didn't expand on his overall health but it was obvious that he hated being fat. His self-loathing is evident in his rant on 'the oleaginous' followed by the story of his own struggle with weight and the lament that, 'Whereas other afflictions enlist the sympathy of our fellow-creatures, this one never fails to be jeered and hooted at, and turned into ridicule by the coarse and vulgar of our species.' For thirty-eight years he had been a 'martyr to obesity'.

'From birth up to within the past twelve months,' he wrote, 'I have had the misfortune to be afflicted with the most dreadful disease that flesh is heir to. It is one that entails suffering both to the body and mind, and from which a vast proportion of humanity suffers in a more or less aggravated form. It is a slow and insidious disease, that never decreases of its own accord, but on the contrary develops itself with one's increasing years, as surely as the most virulent cancer.' At age eighteen he weighed 18 stone so he was aware, from personal experience, 'how fat people catch at every straw to evade a "regimen", and invariably say, as I did, "Nothing will make me thin"; "I've tried everything"; "It's natural in our family"; "My father weighed nineteen stone", &c., &c.'. To these people he wished to say 'Rubbish!' He didn't give a damn if your father weighed 40 or your grandmother 50 stone, he would, he promised, 'GUARANTEE TO REDUCE YOU, perceptibly and with PERFECT SAFETY, if you'll guarantee to follow my instructions'.

Advice to Stout People carried dubious adverts, too, like the one on the inside cover page for alcohol aimed at 'STOUT PEOPLE'. The 'Fifty Dozen of Pure, Genuine Johannisberg Schlosslage, vintage 1868 … is particularly recommended to Stout People by the most eminent Physicians; it takes out the watery substance from the fat and puts sinews in its place'. As well as being blasé about recommending booze, D— S— gave short shrift to those who warned that smoking was 'injurious to the corpulent … this I consider sheer nonsense'. He himself smoked 'from morning to night, and on the contrary believe that it makes up for the larger amount of food one had previously been in the habit of consuming. In America, where I spent many happy years, I was never without "a smoke"' (and it's true that the tobacco companies would soon be exploiting the appetite-suppressing effects of cigarettes in an alarmingly brutal way). The tenor of this short but emphatic pamphlet was of self-loathing, denial, indulgence and punitive correction. Always be very strict with yourself, it said; take no liberties with your diet but don't deny yourself the pleasures of drinking and smoking.

D— S— had tried every remedy for fifteen years, with no results, until he took his own advice and, from 25 November 1881 when he weighed 19 st 13 lb, he lost eighteen inches of girth and 7 st 9 lb in weight so that by 1 October 1882 he was just 12 st 4 lb. While he couldn't produce 'testimonials from a corpulent clergyman in Australia who weighed forty stone and now only fourteen … nor from the fat Countess de Quackador of Buenos Ayres, who attributes her recovery to the sole use of ——' he could produce himself, and he offered to give personal inter-views to corpulent people as a living demonstration of how to lose weight. Investing in a cheap set of scales was a good idea for weighing your food as well as yourself, so that 'by degrees this weekly weighing becomes an amusement, and one that increases as your weight decreases'. People were routinely weighed in sur-geries, and scales became increasingly common in people's homes from the beginning of the twentieth century. Using figures lifted from the data of an insurance company, D— S— gave average weight for height measurements as guidance: those who were five feet tall should weigh in the order of 8 st 3 lb, at 5 ft 6 in. – 10 st 7 lb, and at 6 ft – 13 st.

In the late nineteenth century the growing insurance industry

was on the lookout for ways in which to judge their policy appli-
cants; and, while body weight was known to be an indicator of
risk, there was a lack of statistical evidence to show that overweight
people had a higher mortality rate. In 1901, however, Dr Oscar H.
Rogers of the NY Life Insurance Co. reported that the mortality
of the fatter policyholders was greater than those with an average
weight, and in 1908 the Dublin Standard Table of Heights and
Weights, based on a survey of NY Life policyholders, became the
authoritative reference of average weight (the compiler, Louis
Dublin, was a zoologist by profession). This Standard Table concluded that before the age of thirty-five being overweight was
slightly advantageous, but that over thirty-five it became a distinct
disadvantage. Dublin's standard was accepted by the medical profession – as late as 1980 it was remarked that it was accepted as
the 'absolute standard of human normality'. The involvement of
insurance companies, in recognising the relationship of mortality
to weight and producing calculations on the base of it, highlights
the role that economics has to play in the issue of obesity.

During the nineteenth century a more scientific approach
to diet and dieting emerged as doctors diversified into special-
isms and consolidated their profession. Research became increasingly well organised as traditional notions about, for example,
the workings of the digestive system, were being challenged
or confirmed. Although this process contested the opinion-
ated quackery and fallacious advice that was available it didn't
entirely displace it, and such practices persisted, with science
often appropriated to lend authority and credibility to spurious
ideas and products.

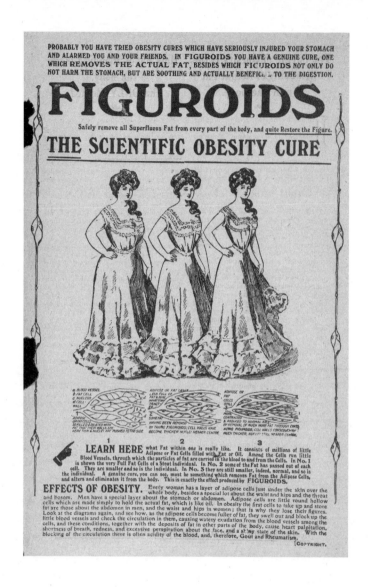

6. Fad diets and crazes, extraordinary apparatus, pummelling, pills, powders, creams and corsets held out the promise of a safe, quick-fix route to a willowy figure – for a price. They have been packed with laxatives and purgatives, and everything from strychnine and lard to washing soda and synthetic hormones. They were pricey, sometimes dangerous, but mostly completely harmless and, of course, useless. The 'fad-promoters' have exploited the insecurities and fears of millions and made the diet industry the monster it is today.

6

Fads and Feeding

FOR HUNDREDS OF YEARS many of us, it seems, have needed someone to worship and emulate, someone whom we'd rather be or at least be like. And there has never been any shortage of icons, from Byron to Greta Garbo to Angelina Jolie, so many of whom have either followed the latest fad or produced and sold their own regimens. Despite the unwholesome recent onslaught of celebrity culture, there have been plenty of examples in the past of this sort of endorsement. The downside of looking up to someone is, of course, being looked down upon, and the distorted, even obsessive, thinking that characterises our relationship with celebrity can, it is said, be traced to the limbic system of our brains. Food, sex and memory are all bedfellows in this system, one of the oldest, most deeply buried structures in the cerebrum, and it is not hard to see how these three fundamental elements become meshed in our perceptions of the celebrities constantly on view. The glimpse of a fat thigh or a double chin before it is airbrushed away can, after all, mean mass denunciation for those trying to elbow their way into the limelight.

An early example of thin celebrity was Elisabeth Amelie Eugenie von Wittelsbach (1837–98), Empress-Consort of Franz

Joseph I, known to the public as 'Sisi'. Lauded as a great beauty, Sisi had developed an extraordinarily strict method of minimising her size as she dealt with state appearances, a growing terror of strangers, timidity, and an intensely critical public gaze. Parallels with Princess Diana are hard to avoid. Sisi was said, unfairly perhaps given her circumstances, to be narcissistic in the extreme. At 5 ft 7 in. tall, quite tall for the time – and taller than her husband – she weighed just 7½ stone. Her waist, which was checked daily by her hairdresser and was emphasised by such tight-lacing that her mother-in-law repeatedly complained about it, had to measure an astonishing nineteen and a half inches or she would refuse to eat.

Sisi married into the royal family in 1854 and flouted convention from the start. She had three pregnancies within four years and her subsequent refusal to eat caused anaemia, greensickness, physical exhaustion and bad nerves. To make herself feel better she took purgatives as well as increasing amounts of exercise with daily, long horse-rides, hours of hiking, and gymnastics (she even had a travelling gym for when she was touring) – all 'sheer foolishness', according to her husband. The Foreign Minister remarked on her 'deepest aversion to any kind of nourishment. She no longer eats anything at all.' Conte Egon Caesar Corti, Sisi's biographer, discussed her poor health in 1860: 'she really is ill, her mental state also affects her body severely. And what would otherwise be a little anaemia, an insignificant cough, under such circumstances, is almost really an illness.' Sisi seemed to improve as soon as she got away from her husband and Vienna.

She spent three hours a day dressing – the lacing alone took an hour – and was said to have had herself sewn into her dresses. She ate only a meagre breakfast, at dinner just a thin broth, and her favourite foods were oranges and milk, one glass a day (she travelled Europe with her own personal cow). As this harsh diet and outdoor activities encouraged wrinkles and weather-beaten skin, she responded by taking even more exercise in the gym with rings, dumb-bells and weights. Her lifestyle was big news in the 1860s and newspapers printed exaggerated stories about her. In 1891, when Sisi was 54 years old, Constantin Christomanos, her Greek Reader, wrote in his diary that, 'This morning before her drive she had me called back to the salon. At the open door between the salon and her boudoir, ropes, bars, and rings were installed. When I saw her, she was just raising herself on the hand-rings. She wore a black silk dress with a long train, hemmed with magnificent black ostrich feathers. I had never seen her so imposing. Hanging on the ropes, she made a fantastic impression, like a creature somewhere between snake and bird.' Her physician diagnosed her as having the telltale breath of an anorexic shortly before she was murdered in Geneva by an anarchist, Luigi Lucheni, who had intended to attack the Duke of Orleans. Instead, Lucheni stabbed the empress as the nearest representative of royalty. Each time he was questioned about his motives he answered, 'Only those who work are entitled to eat.' Such irony.

There was significant nineteenth-century interest, too, on both sides of the Atlantic, in figures such as the medieval Catholic, Catherine of Siena. Her spiritual intensity and fasting were regarded as highly admirable, and relevant to girls in danger of adolescent self-love. The British proto-feminist, Josephine Butler, published a biography of Catherine of Siena in 1879, and Vida Scudder, Wellesley College Professor of English, published her letters in 1895. Anorexia, estimated now to affect about four women in every thousand, was categorised in the nineteenth century by Queen Victoria's doctor, Sir William Gull. In 1895, the *Lancet* reported the case of a starving sixteen-year-old Bristol schoolgirl, who was kept immobile in a hospital bed by wrapping her limbs and body in cotton wool to elevate her body temperature and restrict any activity. She was fed pulverised food every four hours and was refused visits from her family, especially her mother who was forcibly kept away. The girl eventually died, weighing just forty-nine pounds, and hers was the first reported death from the modern disorder of anorexia in English-language medicine, though the condition was then something of a mystery to medicine. The *British Medical Journal* began to cover similar cases, including the 'Amazing Fasting Welsh Girls', and in 1889 the popular press picked it up when the *Boston Globe* ran a story, 'Who Took the Cold Potato? Dr Mary Walker Says the Fasting Girl Bit a Doughnut', on a girl called Josephine Bedard and how she was caught by her doctor allegedly eating in secret.

Medical authority as an agent of social criticism is familiar to us today, from newspapers to television and websites. Doctors Daniel G. Brinton and George H. Napheys, in *The Laws of Health in Relation to the Human Form* published in 1871, had come up with some spurious directives, all bound up with what supposedly looked right: 'The precise medium between corpulence and leanness is hard to attain and harder to keep, so that if this matter attracts a good deal of attention, it is nothing more than right, aesthetically speaking, that it should,' they wrote. This body fascism was, unsurprisingly, hardest on women as 'women are now young longer than they are beautiful', so ought to work hard or face the misery of being thought unattractive.

In the 1890s most American women were looking to Sarah Tyson Rorer (1849–1937) for advice on 'reducing'. Rorer believed that 'an excess of flesh is to be looked upon as one of the most objectionable forms of disease, and must be treated as such'. She was a prolific food writer and journalist, having published fifty-four cookbooks and a regular kitchen column for *Ladies' Home Journal*, but she was no medic. Still, she thought she knew a disease when she saw one, and fat fitted the bill – 'for it certainly is a disease [that] creeps on so slowly that the individual becomes thoroughly wedded to the form of life producing it before he realizes his true condition … The whole machinery will be overtaxed, joints will swell, feet will begin to shuffle, and the mind will become inactive.' Abundance must be suppressed and alcohol shunned, as well as potatoes, rice, bread, sweets and most fatty foods. This was diet as medicine; as old as the hills but with fear and anxiety attached. You would not only end up dead, but ugly, objectionable and dead.

Other doctors saw the fat as 'in a sense comical' and all were 'pitiable'. In 1892, F. Dercum of Jefferson Medical College came up with *adiposis dolorosa*, a 'sorrowful miserable or painful fatness'. This disease lingered on in the medical textbooks for the next sixty years, and was said to affect middle-aged women whose appetites were not excessive but whose aches and pains and tiredness were – middle-aged women today might have another word for it. Older women weren't the only ones to be targeted, of course. In 1905 Dr Emma E. Walker, writing in the 'Pretty Girl Papers' section of the *Ladies' Home Journal*, wrote that, 'On the whole it is better to be too thin than too plump, for an excess of fat may cause serious mischief. It makes one heavy and awkward, and finally the "fat walk" – the waddling gait you know so well – develops, and I beg you to avoid this!'

Yet plump flesh could be fashionable and erotic – in some circumstances and only within reason. From the medieval period on, the 'reproductive figure' – fleshy, full, fertile and round – had been the coveted shape. We can see this in the paintings and drawings of Rubens, Rembrandt in the 1600s, and Renoir in the 1800s. The model used by Manet in his 'Olympia' (1863), for instance, was fiercely criticised for not being plump enough to be desirable. But the ideal female body was only rounded enough to properly differentiate it from the taut male body. There was a distinct difference between desirable flesh and unwanted fat. During the nineteenth century, society's opinions and often unforgivingly harsh judgements on looks, behaviour and morals – particularly women's – had become increasingly vocal. This was the age of the birth of self-help, yet humiliation was never far away as a motivational force.

The eye-catching fascination of fat on show was good business in the nineteenth century in more ways than one. Hugely fat people were then, as now, under the cultural microscope. Massaging away the fat, pounding it out from between the tissues, was popular at the end of the century (and would continue to be so, off and on). George Burwell perfected his obesity belt, the Boston Bon-Contour, in 1892, a contraption that had 100 to 150 electrically charged magneticore discs sewn between lengths of denim, satin and medicated flannel. In 1898 the 'Admiral' Soap Syndicate of London issued a pamphlet, a 'scientific exposition', entitled *The Treatment of Local Obesity by a New Process*, about a medicated soap which would reduce adipose tissue, described as being on the borderline of pathology, on the hips, belly and chin, particularly of women. This sort of fat could, it warned, invade the internal organs, especially the heart and kidneys. Claiming that rubbing the soap on a selected limb would produce a noticeable effect after a fortnight, it promised that after another month a leg given this treatment would diminish by a few inches. The procedure did not recommend a sudden and violent change of regimen, none of these fad methods did, as weightloss with no effort was their major selling point.

In terms of fads, the 'medical idol of the moment' was, according to the *Lancet*, one Horace Fletcher (1849–1914). In American entrepreneurial fashion, Fletcher, 'The Great Masticator', was a man whose revolutionary new diet method was an immense success and a fashionable pastime. 'Fletcherism' promoted an intense kind of mastication: each mouthful of food was chewed until it was liquid and all trace of taste had disappeared – thus

eliminating the risk of 'putrid decomposition' from the gut –
and anything left in the mouth was spat out as not worth the
swallowing. Each mouthful needed a hundred chews at least,
though a shallot, for example, required a little more effort at,
say, 700 chews. Fletcher argued that proper nutrition was the
basis of health and that physical sickness or weakness was down
to shoddy work with your mouth or, as he jauntily put it, your
'three inches of personal responsibility'. One's bowel was also
vitally important and if you chewed well you would defecate less,
and less often. Fletcher himself was quite smug about the fact
that he defecated just once a fortnight, perhaps just managing
two to four ounces, and was happy to report that his waste was
'no more offensive than moist clay' and had 'no more odour than
a hot biscuit'. He always had a sample with him to prove it. At
forty, he had weighed 15 st 7 lb and had been refused life insurance, but by his mid-fifties he was performing physical exercises
like a man half his age, and was described by a nutritionist as a
'physiological puzzle'.

Fletcher's meals consisted of the usual middle-class Edward-
ian fare but in smaller portions, as it was laborious to chew so
long and hard and almost impossible to eat as much. He ate
little meat or really fibrous vegetables for the same reason. Wine
was permitted but must only be swilled around in the mouth.
Fletcher thought little of breakfasting; a piece of toast and a bit
of fruit would do. Oddly, he was a big fan of cereal, eating bowls
of it with full cream milk and lots of sugar, though he doesn't
say what time of day he ate them, and he liked sweets and cakes
and drank sugary coffee. According to Fletcher one could eat
anything one wanted – as long as it was all chewed endlessly and
thoroughly.

If all this sounds slightly left field, so was Fletcher. He had
gone to sea on a whaling vessel in 1864, when he was fifteen, he
had sailed with a crew of Chinese pirates, trained sharpshooters

for the Japanese Army, managed a New Orleans opera company, and eventually made his fortune in San Francisco as a manufacturer of printing ink and an importer of Japanese art before coming up with his big dieting idea. Fletcher was taken very seriously by the medical profession in both America and England and he had many disciples including John D. Rockefeller, Franz Kafka and Henry James. James began by calling him 'the divine Fletcher', but after five years of devoted chewing he had developed a 'sickish loathing' of food. In England, fashionable people were said to hold munching parties, and to time each other with stopwatches to ensure a good five-minute chewing of each forkful of food.

The chewing craze was discussed at length by the British Medical Association, and Professor Michael Foster of Cambridge experimented with it, finding an immediate and very striking effect on the appetite. Fletcher's masticating public became more discriminating, choosing plain foods and finding that they were fully satisfied with less, experiencing, apparently, an increase in their sense of well-being and working powers. Fletcher was examined by Russell H. Chittenden, Professor of Physiology at Yale University, who himself had dieted down from just over 10 stone to 9 stone in 1903 and thought that around two ounces of protein per day for the average man should amply suffice. Fletcher made increasingly grand claims, suggesting social and military uses of his diet system. During the Boer War he advised the British Army in South Africa to try super-mastication so that rations could be reduced by two-thirds, but his idea was rejected, understandably, for political and diplomatic reasons. In 1910, however, after the American and French Armies had tried it, the Royal Army Medical Corps did experiment with Fletcherism but found that the troops needed far more calories than the reduced rations provided and the men all lost weight. In America, Fletcher lent his name to a programme of disease prevention conducted among tramps in Chicago, and in a poverty-stricken area of New York he ran the Kindergarten of Vital Economics where, as well as the three Rs, they taught the three Ms: Munching, Manners and Music. Such experiments shared the classical belief in responsible, civic behaviour, wherein one's eating habits had implications for wider public morality.

Chewing was taken up by popular writers such as George Craston who believed that it was this and not the quality or quantity of food that was important; one shouldn't, he wrote, swallow down food 'like the boa constrictor'. Craston's *Pretty Faces and How They Are Made, Without Paint, Rouges, Cosmetics, or Any Artificial Means: How Everybody Can Be Pretty* (1896), was a diet and beauty book aimed directly at women, and was particularly unpleasant. Alarm bells start to ring when Craston appropriates the supposed laws of nature. A good healthy beautiful body depends, he says, upon one's mode of life, and the 'love of muck and the sweet-tooth of many who clog themselves with toffee, jam, cake, ice-cream, nauseous chip-potatoes, fried fish, &c., nuts, and other indigestible matter, do a great deal of injury to the health of body and mind'. So far so good. Then he continues with: 'The health of the nation is in women's hands, not in the statesman's, nor in the clergyman's, nor the doctor's. The domestic life of women is the key to all!!!' The blows begin to fall. Women who cannot cook or who are bad cooks are hateful and ought to be drowned. 'Seriously speaking,' he writes, 'it would be better for the world and their families if they had a safe journey to heaven and no return ticket!!!'

Not only were women to blame for everyone's ills but they were risking the health of the next generation, too, with their ridiculous vanity: 'there are many fashions, customs and habits which wage war with nature' and one of the worst, for Craston, was tight-lacing, 'which is resorted to until the upper and lower portions of a woman's body are peninsula-fashion connected which gives her the appearance of a giant insect!' No woman who wore tight-laces was fit for motherhood, he raged, 'for she heartlessly cripples and deforms her unborn babe, and ruins her own health by measures of torture worse than any circus-contortionist adopts'. Addressing these bloodless, nervous, irritable women, martyrs to dyspepsia, Craston would say that health and good looks require the 'regular action of every organ of the body, with plenty of room for free motion – no packing, jamming, or pressing of heart, lungs, stomach, &c. One needed room for the blood to flow freely. That would be "pure blood! Pure blood!! Pure blood!!!"'

The state of the nation was emerging as a major political and public concern during this period. The growing eugenics movement was all about good blood and bad, 'improving' the breeding stock of British people, and health, hygiene and beauty were offshoots of these ideas. Bodies were irreversibly damaged by the use of purgatives, wrote Craston, and did great violence to the system, causing cancers, weakening and wearing the body away. No slimming drugs or quack medicines would do any good, he wrote, and he told his readers to 'throw physic to the dogs! throw physic to the dogs!! throw physic to the dogs!!! or down the sink … Better never purchase the nauseous stuff at all! … The ills in your condition are effects! effects!! effects!!!' Craston's rules for a healthy, fit body included chewing your food carefully, wearing flannel next to your skin, getting eight hours' sleep, giving up tea, coffee and fat and, instead, eating home-made wholemeal bread and plenty of vegetables and fruit.

Other popular writers, such James Gross, agreed and spared no one's feelings, calling Americans gluttons, not epicures. 'They swallow, but don't eat; and, like the boa-constrictor, bolt everything, whether it be a blanket or a rabbit … it startles a foreigner to see with what voracity even our delicate women dispose of the infinite succession of dishes on the public tables.' One should not be surprised if meals lasted only three or four minutes. Without conversation, diners bolted their food fast and often, all serious, self-absorbed and silent.

Another commentator noted that women's figures were disguised by the flounces of their frocks so that 'you will hardly be able to distinguish the embonpoint of one of your lady friends from the meagerness of the other'. *Harper's Weekly* suggested that 'these Dresses are very well in their way, but they make us all appear the same size. Why, a Girl might be as thin as a Whipping -post, and yet be taken for a Decent Figure.' The Reverend David Macrae, visiting from Scotland just before the Civil War, said that 'the American girls themselves, I think, are nervous about their thinness, for they are constantly having themselves weighed, and every ounce of increase is hailed with delight ... Every girl knows her own weight to within an ounce or two, and is ready to mention it at a moment's notice. It seems to be a subject of universal interest.' Dr George Beard, in *Eating and Drinking* (1871), had blamed such attitudes on the Calvinist doctrine of cultivated people; they ate little, Beard conjectured, because of the old belief that 'satiety is a conviction of sin'. Meanwhile, the personal columns in American magazines such as *Water-Cure Journal* carried ads from men looking for 'a form medium sized, well developed, erect and plump (not gross, but full and round – I do not admire skeletons)'.

The working of modern civilisation was central to the argument of *Fads and Feeding* (1908) by C. Stanford Read who believed that it brought many undesirable factors, the worst being the rise of the 'fad'. Medicine, he wrote, had made great advances, but where most doctors feared to tread others, with no legitimate authority scientific or otherwise, would inevitably step in to advise the public. These 'fad-promoters' encouraged unnecessary introspection that could be carried too far, 'until it became morbid', and damaged the gullible. People could no longer trust their gut feelings, he argued, because the wear and tear of modern life had overwhelmed them and they were 'full of perverted instincts and cravings ... by no means in harmony with nature'. If everyone blindly followed their instincts life would, he thought, degenerate quickly into chaos as people sought to satisfy their selfish appetites. Stanford Read, like many before him, trembled to think of the world governed by instinct and shuddered to realise that, 'however much they aver to the contrary, there exists a very large section of the community who are nearer living to eat than eating to live'.

To put everyone back on the straight and narrow Stanford Read proposed his 'Common Sense in Diet'. It didn't matter much what one ate, the important point was how much one ate, and how one ate it. Food was necessary to build up and repair waste tissues and to provide energy for work, and the smallest amount of food that would accomplish these ends was the ideal diet. Any surplus was harmful, especially as such surplus would build up over time as one lost sight of cause and effect. No particular foods had to be avoided, but only a very light breakfast was required as well as one really good meal in the evening (almost the reverse of today's common wisdom). Sensible nutrition did not depend upon having 'a pair of scales always at one's elbow' either. He also thought that there were scientific reasons for the idea that a woman needed less nutriment than men, 'even apart from the fact that she is usually of slighter build and usually does not lead such an active life', and he wasn't surprised that some of the fattest women were from the better-off classes. Quoting the psychiatrist Hack Tuke's work on the connection of mind and body, he maintained that the action of the mind was 36 per cent intellect, 56 per cent emotional and 8 per cent will, and people, especially women, should be aware that 'the stomach and the mind cannot be active simultaneously'.

If dieters would just simplify their meals, the great temptation to overeat would be removed. Overeating was, thought Stanford Read, probably as dangerous as excessive drinking. Many agreed, including the influential American psychiatrist, S. Weir Mitchell (1829–1914), who wrote, in *Fat and Blood* (1898), that alcoholism 'gives rise in some people to a vast increase in adipose tissue, and the sodden, unwholesome fatness of the hard drinker is a sufficiently well-known and unpleasant spectacle'. Women were particularly susceptible to morphine, too, which could result in lying about in bed getting fat. Weir Mitchell thought that overeating, laziness and lack of exercise were all too common and he recommended a milk diet (creamless milk for the very fat), although to counteract loss of strength, you could start eating protein foods such as beef, mutton and oysters once the weight had been lost. Bad consequences always came of overeating: 'No one should allow himself to become the subject of obesity as his years advance, and almost invariably it is his own fault if he does.'

The fat under the skin, though it produced discomfort and minimised movement, was not as significant as that within the body which 'clogg[ed] the wheels which should run smoothly'. According to Weir Mitchell, many nervous disturbances were due to this chronic poisoning, including headaches, irritability, depression, drowsiness, lassitude, premature old age and anger, and there was an innate connection between diet and character: 'the avoidance of gluttony, and the simple diet, will always go hand in hand with that which is best in this world, morally, intellectually, and physically'. Stanford Read, however, allowed an exception, believing that a few people were fat because of a 'constitutional taint' and, if this was the case, it was practically impossible to lose weight by any therapeutic means. The average fat person, though, just had to make the effort to diet.

The overweight had to ignore the dangerous advertisements in the public press that praised some new concoction 'which will reduce stoutness in a marvellous degree without any alteration in diet'. The ridiculous idea that losing weight was easy and required no great changes in one's life was nevertheless, he thought, the catch that attracted the 'ever-gullible public'. Using your common sense was the thing: nothing could negate a bad diet or lack of exercise, 'even with the copious perspiration that might accompany it'. The desired weight loss, wrote Stanford Read, would never be achieved in a few weeks or a couple of months – what the dieter needed was a regimen to follow for the rest of his life. And there was no standard, one-size-fits-all diet; one had to take note of personal factors, such as inheritance, and a doctor must treat the patient and not merely the symptoms. A strict habit of temperance would have to be developed so that a sensible attitude to food, drink and mental and physical exercise could be introduced and maintained.

The two objectives of Stanford Read's diet were to reduce the excessive accumulation of fat and to prevent its reaccumulation: the first he considered quite easy, but the second seemed to be made difficult by the dieter's 'want of patience and perseverance'. Half an hour before breakfast the patient must drink a tumblerful of hot or cold water. Breakfast was one to two ounces of toast without butter, some meat – a chop, ham or tongue – a small cup or two of tea or coffee with skimmed milk but definitely no sugar (a sweetener was permitted). A little soup between breakfast and lunch was also allowed if necessary. Lunch consisted of a little cold meat, a small omelette or poached eggs, with some green vegetables, a small crust of bread or toast with a scrape of butter, and one glass of light wine diluted with an equal quantity of water. In the afternoon one could have a cup of tea with skimmed milk but no sugar and a rusk or an unsweetened biscuit. For dinner one might have grilled or boiled fish, but no fatty sauces, or possibly oysters, a little grilled or roasted meat with just a small portion of fat, no potatoes but possibly green vegetables, and for dessert some unsweetened stewed fruit.

One could also take a glass or two of light claret diluted with water, but no whisky, brandy or other spirits. Goose, pork, salmon, eel and mackerel were not allowed as they were far too fatty. An occasional potato was acceptable, and perhaps a little bread, but no dried fruit, thick soups, pastry or sauces. Fluids were limited to thirty ounces and, all in all, it was better to do without alcohol. Climate and season also affected food intake, so that living by the seaside was considered most favourable, for the air and the exercise.

What the dieter must do at all costs is prise the mind away from 'unscientific and illogical self-appointed authorities in the lay-press [who] dogmatise on some diet or particular food'. The more extreme the faddist and their dietary pronouncements, the more the 'converts would rally beneath his standard: and for the sake of novelty, for the sake of belonging to an elect cult, there seem to be an ever increasing number of individuals who for a time, at least, will believe any fresh dietetic rubbish that comes under their notice'. Some faddists might be sincere but most, according to Stanford Read, knew it would bring them the 'kudos and pecuniary compensation' that they were really after at the expense of their gullible customers' health and pockets.

The Salisbury Method, for example, introduced from America at the beginning of the twentieth century, and described in books such as *What Must I Do to Get Well? And How Can I Keep So?*, restricted diet for a time to large quantities of protein only. The Salisbury Method was a descendant of Banting and a precursor of the modern Atkins diet: it limited bread, vegetables and milk in the belief that the dieter would supply the necessary carbohydrates from their own store: 'he consumes his own fat'. To transpose a high-fat diet, such as that of the Arctic, on to urban Americans and Europeans seemed to Stanford Read, for one, like asking for trouble. On the Salisbury Method one could have only rump steak, cod fish and hot water for the first two weeks – as much as three pounds of steak and one pound of cod fish was consumed daily, with six pints of hot water sipped slowly. Later, one could begin to reduce the amount of fluid taken and begin to vary the types of meat. It was acknowledged that this was an extremely difficult regimen to stick to but, of course, according to the patter, 'remarkable results have been obtained'. Recommended as best for those whose fat was due to overeating, it attracted serious criticism, not only from Stanford Read, as possibly causing strain on the kidneys. Indeed similar objections had been made about the renowned Banting system. Overweight people could not dodge the laws of nature, critics warned, and if you overdid things, Nature would remind you but she would never forgive you.

Hormones were all in vogue at this time, too. Early experimental work on these 'new' substances took place in America and Europe during the 1890s and, in the early twentieth century, Edward Sharpey-Schafer (1850–1935) laid down the physiological foundations of endocrinology. Although some considered the theories dubious, and the unreliability of results meant that treatments were regarded as potentially dangerous by many medics – they were still heralded as exciting breakthroughs by the press and public, and by the pharmaceutical companies. Fat, among other bodily mysteries, was now thought to do with hormones and glands, in particular the thyroid. If you were fat and had no success with dieting then perhaps you suffered from Endogenous Obesity, the result of a defect in the internal regulatory system of the body which gave rise to a lack of thyroxine. Iodine, isolated, named and in use by 1813 for thyroid complaints, was now a remedy for excess fat. It was one of the secret ingredients in some of the most popular and widely advertised patent medicines against fat: Allan's Anti-Fat, Frank J. Kellogg's Safe Fat Reducer, Dr Bertha C. Day's Fort Wayne prescriptions, Marmola, Newman's Obesity Cure, Chichester's Corpus Lean, Rengo, Dr Gordon's Elegant Pills, Corpulin, Elimiton, Phy-th-rin, San-Gri-Na, Trilene tablets – all these contained either fucus (bladderwrack) or thyroid extract, or Ipecac (a plant-based emetic), camphor (an appetite suppressant), potassium acetate (a diuretic) and digitalis (a stimulant).

By the 1920s the medical profession considered the warnings given about women's dieting habits as part of the Progressive Era's preventive medicine programme: 'unwise and fanatical' diets and a 'mania for thinness' were a new perceived threat to health, and doctors began to attack what they considered to be quasi-scientific diets – regimens of lemon juice, milk and bananas, special breads, seaweeds and the patent medicines, as well as bath powders, pastes and thinning salts.

Dr W. W. Baxter came up with Phytoline which he said upgraded fatty tissue to muscle; he had seen it used as a reducing agent for plump migatory birds. Slenderine and an accompanying weight-loss programme was produced by Hattie Beal & Co. who received more than two hundred letters a day after it was advertised with the slogan: 'You at once become master of your own body. You CONTROL your weight ever after.' The advertisements for these products were plastered across America, coast to coast, and their brand names hid basic ingredients: arsenic, which speeds up the system, was an ingredient in some slimming drugs, often mixed with strychnine, caffeine and phytolacca or pokeberry (a common emetic and purgative); Berledets was made of boric acid, corn starch and milk sugar; Human Ease had sodium bicarbonate and lard (!); Densmore's Corpulency Cure was sassafras tea; Lucile Kimball's Powder was a mixture of red pepper, menthol, bitters, aloes, soap, Epsom salt and washing soda.

Lucile advertised her product with friendly commiseration, 'Everything you ever tried, I tried,' she said in 1914. 'I went through exercises, rolled on the floor, cut down my food, gave up candy, fats and starches, wore elastic clothing, tried electricity, massage, osteopathy, vibration, hot and vapor baths, swallowed pellets, capsules and tea – gained as rapidly as I lost.' She sold her nonsense in pink and brown tablets and as a bath powder. Doctors endorsed weight control but worried about the desire for a 'barber-pole figure', which they believed was gaining ground after the Great War and into the 1920s.

An advert for Figuroids effervescing tablets appeared in the February 1908 issue of the *Windsor Magazine*, an illustrated monthly for men and women, and showed a young woman in before and after modes. It rubbished other anti-fat products: 'Probably you have tried obesity cures which have seriously injured your stomach and alarmed you and your friends,' it said, but Figuroids were a 'genuine cure' which completely removed 'actual fat', did no harm, were soothingly beneficial to the digestion, and would 'quite restore the figure'. Every woman, it went on, had a 'layer of adipose cells just under the skin over the whole body, besides a special lot about the waist and hips and about the throat and bosom', and men had a special layer about their abdomens, all of which robbed them of a youthful figure. The images revealed just 'what FAT within one is really like', a sure-fire way to arouse disgust and self-loathing. Look at the diagrams again, the advert demanded, and see how the fat cells invade your body, swell up and block up blood vessels causing heart palpitation, shortness of breath, redness, excessive perspiration about the face, and a shiny state of the skin. Who wouldn't want to buy a pill and stop all that fat from being carried in the blood to and from the cells, spreading like a plague throughout one's body?

While English women were tucking into Figuroids and American women were rolling on the floor twenty times in loose clothing before they missed their breakfasts, and again, twenty times after their evening lemon juice, the men were not being left behind. Frenchmen were flocking to Dr Jean Alban Bergonié whose method involved sitting in a reclining chair with electrodes fixed to the back and seat. The patient sat with other electrodes on wet towels over his thighs, under his legs, across his abdomen and arms, all held in place with rubber bracelets and bags of sand. Dr Bergonié then passed a current of 50 milliamperes through the whole shebang to contract his patient's muscles a hundred times a minute, a charge sufficiently powerful to raise the body, even under eighty-eight pounds of sand. Bergonié claimed that a one-hour sitting was the equivalent of a ten-mile run in a heavy sweater, and all that 'without the intervention of the will, and almost without sensation, the patient being occupied during the treatment with his own thoughts or with the book he is reading'.

In America, the first reducing salon opened in Chicago in 1914 and was equipped with Gardner Reducing Machines that enveloped male clients in two sets of adjustable rollers. Women could get rolled at W. F. Taylor's Corset Shop in San Diego and at the Bush Sanatorium in Louisville. Some machines featured an electrical ring roller with helical springs of tempered steel and rollers mounted on ball bearings that could squeeze up and down your body eighty times per minute. The laziness and quick-fix lack of effort of these mechanical pummellers was derided by the occasional lone voice, such as the *North American Journal of Homeopathy* which, in 1910, meekly suggested that 'Corpulency should not be met by a so-called short cure ... the cure should last as long as life and should merely consist in putting the muscles to their natural use.' This advice disappeared beneath all the adverts for slimming potions and devices.

In *Rational Hydrotherapy* (1900) John Harvey Kellogg pre-scribed water cures for obesity, including cold rain douches, sweating packs, cold dripping sheets, short plunge baths and electric arc light baths. His sanitarium had vibrating chairs and platforms, trunk rollers, chest beaters and stomach beaters for exercising and massaging the overweight, who were rapidly becoming his main customers: more than 7,000 patients a year were using his spa facilities by the 1920s. In addition to all the pummelling and water cures, they were treated to enemas and a low-calorie, high-bulk, moderate protein diet. A clean and lean diet, together with lots of water and yoghurt administered from both ends, would also, Kellogg believed, help with sexual excess. Kellogg was a religious man and the sanitorium where he was chief medical officer was owned by the Seventh Day Adven-tist Church. He was also a surgeon specialising in repair of the sphincter and wanted to extend the 'sensitive colon conscience' to the habits of daily living. He admired Fletcher and his mas-tication theory and helped him to organise the Health and Effi-ciency League of America.

During the nineteenth century, fad dieting had really begun to take off, as older weight-loss remedies, such as an infusion of thrift (or sea-pink, a coastal plant), had begun to lose ground both to more sensational ideas, and to science. The way people lived and their attitudes to body size were changing. In Europe and America, as people moved away from the fields and into urban environments in order to work in the growing industries for a higher disposable income, they began to eat higher-calorie refined foods such as white bread, sugary fancies and attractively packaged fast fried meals. More and more working-class people were becoming overweight where once excess fat had been regarded as a middle- and upper-class problem.

Weight loss demanded – as everyone was beginning to recognise through an ever more visible media – constraint, compulsion, discipline and submission. *Atlantic Monthly* carried a description of a woman trying on dress she had not worn for a year: 'The gown was neither more or less than anticipated. But I ... the fault was on me ... I was more! Gasping I hooked it together. The gown was hopeless, and I ... I am fat.' One answer to her problem was aired in the *English Woman's Domestic Magazine* which printed letter upon letter on corsetry and tight-lacing (alongside, it has to be said, those on boarding schools and fetishistic sado-masochism): 'Well applied restraint is in itself attractive' and 'half the charm in a small waist comes, not in spite of, but on account of, its being tight-laced – the tighter the better'.

This penchant applied to men, too. In a piece called 'A Male Wasp Waist' which appeared in the *Family Doctor* in 1886, the writer admired women's waists and confessed that he, too, wore a corset, 'like a lady', and had 'been struck by the number of men who have admired me, and would, no doubt, have liked to put their arms round my small waist'. Men in corsets were nothing new: dandyism in Regency England had practically demanded the wearing of such garments – George Cruikshank's satirical prints of men in stays included 'Laceing a Dandy' in 1819, wherein the servant says, 'If you don't pull tight, my Lord will have a damn big John Bull belly', and the vain, fat Joseph Sedley in Thackeray's *Vanity Fair* had tried 'every girth, stay, and waistband then invented'. Sensibilities and fashions changed, of course, and after about 1850 men who wore corsets said they did so only for support or for medical reasons.

In the 1880s advertisements in magazines pictured small girls in corsets in special 'healthy' models designed for immature bodies, and sold apparently for the purpose of correcting slovenliness and a crooked posture; they were no longer regarded as erotic and evil as they had been in the sixteenth century. In the late nineteenth century corsets for girls were effective in maintaining ideals of femininity and nipping girls into shape early on. It may be that our perspective now is not unlike that of the early modern period; portents of sexuality in the young are regarded with disquiet today, as made clear by recent anxieties about fashions aimed at pre-adolescents.

A more troubling aspect of the manipulating of bodies could be read between the lines. It wasn't just the fat who wore corsets, this opportunity was open to all, as an advert for Evans and Bale of London's 'Ideal Corset' showed. This item, an early version of today's silicone gel bra-inserts, or 'chicken fillets', would apparently perfect a 'thin bust'. Indeed, 'Words cannot describe its effect in perfecting thin figures. Softly padded Regulators (Patented) inside each breast, laced more or less closely; regulate at the wearer's pleasure any desired fullness, with their graceful curves of a beautifully proportioned bust.' But it was mainly the plumper person who purchased. 'I am very stout, I should look like a tub without a corset,' ran one complaint in Helen Ecob's *Well-Dressed Woman* (1893), and she replied, 'It is no worse to look like a tub than an hourglass ... your size will be less apparent if your clothing is loose. Of the two evils choose the less. Obesity can never be made becoming; if it can not be overcome, it must be accepted as one accepts other physical deformities.'

A self-proclaimed 'beauty expert', Henry Fink, who wrote *Romantic Love* in 1887, insisted that 'There is one horror which no lady can bear to contemplate, viz. Fat', and 'many women consider the corset necessary as a figure-improver, especially if they suffer from excessive fatness'. But they were wrong, said Fink. That fat was bad was true, but it shouldn't be squeezed and contained, it should be burned away through respiration, and corsetry impeded that function. In fact, the corset was, he argued, one of the principal causes of women's corpulence: it actually made you fatter because, over the course of time, the downward pressure of the garment distended the abdomen which became more flabby due to atrophy of the back and abdominal muscles. Dr Anna M. Galbraith, writing in *Hygiene and Physical Culture for Women* (1895), also bemoaned the way corsets interfered with breathing and forced the wearer into a sedentary life simply because exercise was impossible while one was strapped into such an unforgiving piece of underwear.

Still, in the anonymously penned *Beauty* (1890), the author was certain that, despite the criticism, most women would continue to wear their corsets for centuries to come. There were, you see, women whose figures required support and who, without aid of this kind, were rendered extremely uncomfortable to themselves and 'beyond question, unsightly to others', these 'possessors of bulky figures would suffer both physically and mentally' without their corsets. In Europe, however, this suffering didn't seem to concern women quite so much even though the sheath-like 'Hip-Confiner' or 'Thigh-Diminishing' corsets were built of reinforced cloth and steel. In 1901 the *Lady's Magazine* reported excitedly on a new corset that was all the rage in Paris. This new, straight-fronted garment would catch on quickly, they thought, and was likely to create a new style of waist and figure – the bust could drop down a bit and the belly had to be kept flat. A *Vogue* Paris correspondent noted that 'the fashionable figure is growing straighter and straighter, less bust, less hips, more waist, and a wonderfully long, slender suppleness about the limbs ... How slim, how graceful, how elegant women look!' But the messages were mixed – in 1902 *Vogue* was proclaiming that 'to judge by the efforts of the majority of women to attain slender and sylph-like proportions, one would fancy it a crime to be fat'.

Thinness triumphed, though, at least in Europe, according to the *Journal des Dammes et des Modes* in 1912, and 'Your glances no longer go to anyone but the willowy, slender woman ... It is no longer a question of breasts or hips ... I challenge you to notice a fat woman today, so much has the tyranny of fashion imperiously formed and strangled our preferences ... Nothing rejuvenates likes thinness, and ... youth is a priori thin.' By 1922 *Vogue* was wondering whether, 'with the aid of the corsetiere, the physical culturist and the non-starchy diet, shall we soon develop a race of slender, willowy women?', after all, life was much more enjoyable for the slim and active, and an excess of *avoir dupois* meant inactivity and boredom. Fashion pundits insisted that 'Stout women must wear corsets to hold their flesh' which could then be more attractively and evenly distributed about the body. Rubber corsets were too feeble: 'She who must struggle with heavy flesh is not wise to permit herself the comfortable pleasure of rubber corsets' which allowed the fat to spread. What she needed instead was 'strongly knit surgical elastic'. But according to Anne Rittenhouse in *The Well-Dressed Woman* (1924), rubber corsets were best because they had the 'merit of reducing the thick flesh over the waist by friction', and you could exercise in them. By 1935 American *Vogue* was reporting that 'there is no more important purchase in a woman's wardrobe than her corset'.

In the quest to lose fat, the overweight increasingly became slaves to the recycled, quick-fix and rogue ideas that just might help them get thin again. Fashions and methods, fuelled by scientific advance, changed depending on the times and there were now plenty of outlets to spread the message. And, just like today, fad diets and ineffectual advice were continually remodelled and promoted as though they were brand new. Body-shaping and weight awareness became popular interests in a way they had not been before, as men and women avidly read the proliferating magazines and newspapers, began to scrutinise the new pin-ups, and internalise the idea of weight-watching. Films had taken up the message – in 1920 the popular Fatty Arbuckle, playing Sheriff

'Slim' Hoover in the film *The Round-Up*, wailed that 'Nobody loves a fat man', while politician Thomas B. Reed opined that 'No gentleman ever weighs more than 200 pounds.' Dieting and body shape have always been political issues, both personal and public. The subject of weight was never merely an individual concern, and during this period it became even more of a social phenomenon.

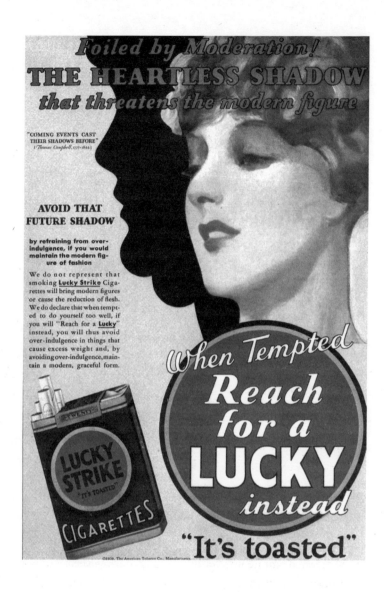

7. A whole series of the American Tobacco Company's Lucky Strike cigarette adverts were a part of the 'indoctrination of the nation' into diet-mania. In the early to mid-twentieth century cynical commercial interests in the diet business exploded. Humiliation and gullibility were ruthlessly exploited to push faddish, easy, fast weight-loss methods promising that you could eat what you liked and not have to work hard or suffer for the ideal figure.

7

Keep Your Eyes Open and Your Mouth Shut

THE DAWNING OF THE AGE of slenderness, which we inhabit fully today, began in the 1920s with the fashion of the Flapper girls after the First World War – it was quite the thing to be flat-chested and boyish when there were so few boys left. Allied propaganda during the war had portrayed German women as fat and frumpy and, by 1918, the message was that 'there is one crime against the modern ethics of beauty which is unpardonable; far better it is to commit any number of petty crimes than to be guilty of the sin of growing fat'. After the Great War it was the French who were setting the trends in body shape; in the pre-war period the *modiste* Paul Poiret had come up with a fashion style he called *le vague*, a loose way of dressing which eliminated the waist, hips and bum in favour of a high-waisted, small-breasted empire line, and these long, narrow sheath tunics were popular well into the 1920s along with the new, rubber girdles that held everything in.

In 1922, Jeanne Lanvin's chemise, a straight frock with a simple bateau neckline, was transformed by Chanel into a Flapper's uniform, with a waistline dropped to the hips, showing more leg and a smoother silhouette. Beneath these, women wore flattening bras constructed of shoulder straps and a single band of material that encased the whole torso, and these French styles were soon taken up by the burgeoning American ready-to-wear market. A Parisian doctor was sufficiently interested to remark that, 'Nowadays it is not the fashion to be corpulent; the proper thing is to have a slight, graceful figure far removed from embonpoint, and a fortiori from obesity. For once, the physician is called upon to interest himself in the question of feminine aesthetics.'

The hordes of single women, their lives and horizons changed by war, provided rich pickings for the diet business, the new fashions giving a wonderful stimulus to that branch of charlatanry that involved 'anti-fat' products. So wrote Arthur J. Cramp, in his essay, 'Fooling the Fat' (1928). Cramp had nothing but contempt for quack remedies, 'With the possible exception of the credulity of the bald-headed man in the field of hair-growers,' he wrote, 'there is nowhere to be found such simple trustfulness in the veracity of printer's ink as that possessed by the obese within the realm of fat cures'. Women in particular, he thought, ate badly, exercised little, and wanted a quick-fix panacea to transform them from 'stylish stout' to lissom 'boyish form'. Their ignorant and naive belief that 'science should make it possible for human beings to violate physiological laws with impunity explains why those shrewd individuals who put out "anti-fats" nearly always emphasise the claim that when using their products or devices: there is no need for hard work, and no need to diet.'

Examples of early twentieth-century advertising suggest that weight-watching women were insistently targeted. Advertisements from the 1920s and 1930s for the American Tobacco Company cigarettes, Lucky Strikes, ran with 'Reach for a Lucky instead of a Sweet.' Some were yet more explicit. One shows a thin young woman with a shadow of a fat, double-chinned face lurking behind her – 'THE MENACING SHADOW that threatens the modern figure!' it says, and 'WARN HER 'ere her bloom is past.' But the widely held belief that smoking helps keep you thin, cynically exploited in early cigarette advertising, has recently been shown to have its basis in fact. In 2011, litigation documents revealed that the tobacco giants Philip Morris and American Tobacco had, in fact, added appetite suppressants to their cigarettes and that four other companies had at least tested substances with similar potential, including amphetamine and nitrous oxide, better known as laughing gas. The documents, which date from 1949 to 1999, show that the industry has exploited dieters for over fifty years in an effort to convince people that smoking can turn you into Kate Moss (even though we know that if you acquire a fag habit you could finish up skinnier than you ever anticipated). According to the *European Journal of Public Health*, this could show why smokers who give up the habit so often gain weight. The number of women smokers increased dramatically during the 1940s and 1950s, and female smokers are still vulnerable to the suggestion that there is a weight-control benefit to the habit. A recent study in the journal *Tobacco Control* of 500 young women found that those who came across female-oriented packaging – super-skinny cigarettes half the depth of a normal pack and branded with words such as 'slim' and 'vogue' – were more likely to think that smoking equals thin.

Women were castigated for being too fat, thinking about being too fat, trying to diet, eating too much, feeding their families badly, for vanity and ignorance. Dr Cecil Webb-Johnson, author of *Why Be Fat?* (1923), treated his predominantly female patients with a patronising slickness. He promised them that they could lose several stones in weight and look twenty years younger. The doctor's clientele, unlike Banting's some sixty years before, were wealthy and he had his eye on their luxurious, sedentary lifestyles as well as on their purses. He instructed them not to get into a handy passing bus if they only had to go from

Piccadilly Circus to Burlington House; they should jolly well walk the short distance. Greed is craving beyond the satisfaction of need, according to Webb-Johnson, who had become interested in dietetics and disorders of metabolism while serving as a major and a medical officer in Calcutta during the First World War (he was also well known, says his obituary, as a composer of waltz tunes and other light musical pieces). His directions for dealing with what he scientifically termed (and there's nothing like a scientific turn of phrase to instill confidence and deference) 'over-adiposity', were to cut back on fluids, and to eat natural, seasonal foods. So, for a summer dinner, Webb-Johnson recommended broiled smelts (a 'good-looking small fish'), or veal and cabbage, while in autumn you could dine on oysters, boiled beef and cabbage, stewed apples and mushrooms on toast.

He also identified specific fat-forming foods that women must deny themselves. To our modern eyes some seem well chosen, but others quite random. The idea of starchy foods as dangerously fat-forming was well known, so Webb-Johnson issued a resounding NO to cereals, starches such as spaghetti, vermicelli and macaroni, and all the 'so-called breakfast foods', pastry, cakes, puddings and pies. Neither should they let potatoes, carrots, beets, parsnips, peas or beans pass their lips, nor figs, dates, raisins, currants or mulberries – all full of sugars. Milk, sugar, butter, cheese, jam, honey and marmalade were forbidden, as were all beers and sweet wines, and any liqueurs or sweetened mineral waters such as ginger beer, ginger ale and lemonade. This was a low-carbohydrate, low-sugar diet, but it was also low in fats and proteins, and meats such as pork were considered very bad on this score. So too were ham, bacon, goose, duck and fat meat of any kind, as well as salmon, mackerel, eels, pilchards, sardines, kippers, bloaters, crab and lobster. It must have been very hard to find anything to eat that Webb-Johnson really approved of.

The 'unlovely condition of corpulence' that Dr Leonard Williams mercilessly described in *Obesity* (1926) marked out as contemptible those whose bodies revealed 'self-indulgence, greed, and gormandising', most of whom were 'disgusting because they represent an unsightly distortion of the human form divine, and a serious impairment of the intellectual faculties'. Or, loosely translated, the fat were little more than stupid and unacceptable, and they had a duty to go on diets in order keep everybody else from being offended at the sight of them. The fat, in short, were selfish. Obsessive dieters were little better: no man, Williams opined, had any right to be really fat; no woman had any right to be really thin. Overeating was not only a gross luxury during these straitened post-war times, it was also a great personal mistake.

In *Dietotherapy* (1918) Dr William Edward Fitch made it quite clear that this and 'the taking of improper food' gave rise to a great variety of diseases, especially in individuals who had hereditary tendencies to certain maladies. Occasional overeating might not hurt, he wrote, but when carried on as habit one could expect to get fat and get ill. It produced biliousness, in which the stomach and intestines were gorged, the tongue heavily coated, the bodily secretions altered in composition and, finally, the nervous and muscular systems were depressed. This worrying combination of conditions would lead to physical as well as mental depression, for 'an overfed boiler soon burns out, it flues become choked with ashes which accumulate faster than they can be removed'.

Such stern edicts may have seemed positively generous when compared to Dr William Leonard and his Unfired diet. This one was just as it sounds: 'only those foods which are uncooked are suitable'. You were to restrict your meals to the following:

1. Dairy Produce: eggs, milk, cream, butter, cheese, cream cheese; honey in moderation.

2. Uncooked Vegetables: lettuce, endive, chicory, mustard and cress, watercress, cucumber, radish, tomato, spring onion, corn salad, dandelion, celery, young cabbage, carrots, turnips, artichokes, and parsnips sliced very thin or grated.
   (Any condiments were allowed, as was a dressing made with raw eggs, milk, mustard, pepper, oil, and vinegar or lemon juice, though salt should be used sparingly.)
3. Uncooked Fruits: apples, pears, bananas, oranges, grapes, strawberries, raspberries, blackberries, peaches, nectarines, green figs. Dried fruits were considered not very valuable, but there was no objection to figs, prunes or dates.
4. Oysters, uncooked, and caviar.

Butcher's meat, boiled puddings, cakes, chocolates and sweets were absolutely out of the question, including fructose-rich fruits. This diet had a serious laxative effect, what with the fresh greens, the use of cooking water, raw fruits between meals and the advice that figs made a handy snack when out and about. Boiled oranges, prunes, nuts and oils, Leonard said, were extremely effective, as was half a teaspoonful of olive oil several hours before or after meals, or oil mixed with lemon or orange juice or as emulsion with milk. Paraffin oil, too, could be swallowed or spread on crackers. In 1917, however, the *Journal of the American Medical Association* carried a protest letter from Dr Harold Gifford: 'An oil enema is so elaborately disagreeable a function that I often wonder how many of the men who light-heartedly order their patients to inject half a pint of olive oil every night for a year or so have tried it themselves.' Still, everything one ate had to be raw, according to Leonard, and it all had to be chewed remorselessly. There was work to be done here, almost as an austere form of punishment for any previous sinful behaviour at the table. Dr Leonard told his patients to 'keep your eyes open and your mouth shut', advice that was probably already familiar to most women of the period.

Dr Eustace Chesser (1902–73) was more even-handed in his attitudes to the sexes. Chesser was a modern, radical thinker who wrote *Slimming for the Million* in 1939 (so free-thinking was he, in fact, that his next book, *Love Without Fear,* on sexual technique, landed him in court on an obscenity charge in 1942). Chesser was another low-carb, high-protein advocate who argued that 'it is not so much the quantity of food you eat, as what you eat', in which calorie intake was not as important as the amount of fat-forming food consumed. To start the day, he advised a glass of hot water or tea without sugar, with a grapefruit and lean bacon and eggs for breakfast; vegetable soup, a satisfying portion of lean meat and 'over-ground' vegetables, and fresh fruit for lunch; and then, 'where habit dictates, a cocktail can proceed dinner', which meal should be similar to lunch, perhaps substituting fish for meat. All sugars 'should be avoided like the devil!', especially chocolates which are one of 'obesity's biggest allies' and 'a constant temptation to ladies'.

Chesser's sensible approach was sympathetic and realistic; he was aware that the overweight could be sensitive, but would want to eat a relatively ordinary if low-carb diet. His advice follows on from Banting's which in turn directly informs diets such as *Dr Atkins' Diet Revolution* (1972) and, more recently, the Dukan diet. Indeed, it has been said of the Atkins diet that its sheer monotony and simplicity, ruining a dieter's appetite, was what made it successful – a well-tried concept. But having no appetite was still, perhaps, preferable to being just 'an abundance of fat'. In 1930 Helena Rubinstein damned fat as 'something repulsive' in her book *The Art of Feminine Beauty*. Fat was not, in her influential opinion, 'in accord with the principles that rule our conception of the beautiful'. This new idea that a slim boyish body was more feminine and sexy than the rounded, womanly shape was certainly a departure from the traditional norm, but it was in accord with some post-war attitudes that regarded working women as lesser females, women without those 'characteristics that marked her out as only for childbearing'.

But the medical profession, in the shape of the President of the American Medical Association, Wendell C. Phillips, implored young women not to blindly follow beauty ideals that endangered their health and even their chances of motherhood – still regarded in most quarters as a woman's primary purpose. Fashionable Flappers of the time, according to a doctor who spoke at the world's first Adult Weight Conference convened by the American Medical Association in New York in 1926, had 'mastered the art of eating their cake and yet not having it, inducing regurgitation, after a plentiful meal, either by drugs or mechanical means'. Such women also went in for high colonic irrigations, cathartics and lots of iodine. The medical profession was horrified to a man by the preposterous foolishness of it all. 'Is there no humbug too raw to feed the fat?' wondered those at the conference, which had been called, ironically, to determine standards of weight in a painstaking search for the 'normal'. All agreed, however, in condemning the fad diet craze and the barber-pole figure. American women, the medics complained, had pounded, dieted and drugged themselves, and submitted to tortures rivalling those of the inquisition, and all in the search for beauty. And all – the young and the old, the long and the short – were apparently trying to pour themselves into the same mould, all in search of the same tiny body.

Dr Morris Fishbein (1889–1976), whose first diet book, *Your Weight and How to Control It* (1929) (a scientific guide by medical specialists and dieticians), was published following the New York conference, was appalled by 'The Craze For Reducing'. Fishbein, an editor of the *Journal of the American Medical*

Association was an influential man and, with the arrogance of a medical professional in a deferential society, he bemoaned the increased public knowledge of calories and vitamins, exercise, massage, electrical apparatus and thyroid extracts. But he had a point: the problem rested, he wrote, with the burgeoning diet industry and its indoctrination of the nation's women. Newspapers, magazines and billboards were 'deluged with advertisements of nostrums of varying efficiency and danger'. There were intricate electric manipulating or vibrating devices especially for women (dual-purpose), and chewing gums containing dangerous drugs were distributed on the streets! Phonographic records were developed for systematic exercises that were taken without regard to the physical condition of the person concerned. Even the radio spouted calisthenics to which women rolled or somersaulted on the floor in an attempt to rid themselves of what they thought was superfluous poundage. 'Any woman you ask,' he wrote, 'can tell you the relation between weight and good looks. Thousands of women – and many men – study the scales each morning with the same passionate interest that Wall Street gives to the stock quotations.'

Fishbein speculated as to whether the changes in women's fashion were responsible for the diet craze or vice versa – he was concerned that, by leaving off their corsets, women were trying to control their fat by other potentially dangerous means. Textbooks of hygiene had increasingly dwelt on the damage corsets could do to one's liver and on the gross distortion of one's figure but, he believed, fashions had improved greatly long before the mania for thinness had come to so disturb the nation. Logical as it may have seemed to think that the figure to which the clothes were fitted was what actually controlled the styles, 'a study of the styles seems to indicate that women have always been unreasonable in adapting the physical body to the styles and permitting the necessities of existence to make the best of it'. Women were not the same the world over, he cautioned, and the American girl was an end product of a mixture of races, predominantly Anglo-Saxon. She was usually somewhat thin, often rather angular, and not infrequently awkward and it is clear that Fishbein felt she had become corrupted somehow, had grown past her plump and feminine best, become nervous and deviant through the old anxiety-inducing idea of over-civilisation.

Dieting robbed women of their femininity, he thought, and not only that, it sent the press into a frenzy of fear over a broken society, rife with lesbianism, even as that same press reaped the rewards of ads for a slew of dieting products and devices. Of all the fads that had afflicted mankind, none seemed to Fishbein more difficult to explain than the desire of American women to be thin. Thin women were not feminine; fat was feminine and the only true badge of womanhood, necessary for successful pregnancy and childbirth. Not only was female fat a physiological necessity, it was a political necessity, and one that American society rested upon. The fad for dieting was nothing less than 'the result of the rise of feminism and the passing of some eleven millions of women out of the home and into industries and occupations which were formerly the prerogatives of men'. As evidence of this feminism Fishbein cited the binding of breasts, the bobbing of hair, and the 'attempt to reduce the figure to male-like slenderness or perhaps the desire for a greater ease of movement required by a change in the natures of women's work'. A woman reduced to the point of malnutrition was, he considered, deeply unattractive, and science must prove it, viewing 'with alarm the present tendency in this country to underestimate the importance of maintaining women as feminine personalities'.

If the male and female norms were undermined by fad dieting it could, he argued, lead to a 'dangerous form of egotism which may eventuate in a disturbance in the social status of the home' and, in fact, 'some specialists in the psychology of sex assert that the tendency in woman to change her form, her mode of dress, and her interests will result in a perversion of sex attraction which may be of the most serious character'. The upending of heterosexuality and the rise of lesbianism! The destruction of the proper order, and all because of dieting. Gentle curves most closely approximated the work of nature, wrote Fishbein and 'the craze for thinness is an attempt to modify the process of nature by means against which nature itself will inevitably revolt'. Fishbein, caught in the panic about women's changing roles, readily conflated culture with nature and tried to back it up with science.

Another American doctor, Harlow Brooks, was anxious to point out that the true 'Price of a Boyish Figure' was a grave risk of irreparable injuries. He scoffed at standardisation – 'we can never be standardized until we are able, as Oliver Wendell Holmes so quaintly said, to "select our ancestors with much greater care"' – and until this might be engineered he warned against fad diets, saying that those who didn't consult a doctor ran health risks including sterility, anaemia, stress, and susceptibility to typhoid, pneumonia, influenza and colds. Brooks thought that there were three types of dieter: young girls; older women who wished to be considered young; and middle-aged men who wanted to increase their business efficiency (!) and were 'anxious to reduce their bay-windows'. Dieting, he continued, might sound harmless but, get this, 'a woman who is naturally sweet-tempered, good-natured, competent, can become transformed into a different person. She becomes petulant, unreasonable, and hard to get along with' and, again, might even end up as a lesbian.

French women, meanwhile, were also getting strong advice on sensible behaviour and dieting. How many of them had died owing to their imprudent use of so-called light-baths, by dry or moist sweatings? How many others had strained their hearts by violent and irrational gymnastics, imposed by quacks possessing no medical knowledge, instead of being prescribed by a competent doctor? Jean Frumusan's *The Cure of Obesity* (1924) berated them soundly for these 'foolish' behaviours and for overeating, particularly of bread, and drinking too much alcohol. These problems affected women across the classes – the well-to-do had an abundance of courses and choice, and the workers in factories or offices were presumably just ignorant. When it came to marriage and fat they were all at fault as most of them came to their wedding weak and anaemic through dieting. This poor specimen of a wife was letting herself in for a wretched, melancholy gestation, a long and painful parturition, and post-confinement consequences which would most likely make her a permanent invalid due to her great accumulation of fat. The life of a married woman was, thought Frumusan, usually less active than that of the single, for when she became a mother her social life dried up, she ate more and more and became a victim of 'matrimonial obesity', and often her poor husband did too. Then, upon realising that she was beginning to thicken, she would tighten her corsets, restrict her diet, and swallow potions recommended by her dressmaker, a friend or a newspaper. Frumusan showed little sympathy for these women, little understanding of their narrow circumstances, and even less faith in their intelligence – they 'become the victim of certain institutions managed by ignoramuses'.

Diet therapy, he fretted, was a chaotic free-for-all. There was a dearth of proper treatments but plenty of contradictory methods, often transmitted from one generation to another, which could not, he thought, stand the feeblest critical examination. The results were always poor and it was difficult to decide which was worse: 'the calm audacity of the lying statements made by those who recommend their wares or the fathomless naïveté of the doctors and the public who adopt them'. Institutes were exploiting fat like merchandise, and far too many theories, fashionable remedies and ingenious clinical discoveries had 'each in turn been praised to the skies, to be subsequently consigned to oblivion'. It was true, wrote Frumusan, that by dint of under-feeding a fat person and extracting all moisture from his or her system, one might occasionally succeed in temporarily melting the space-filling fat, but this only initiated absolute disaster. Publicity had become such a powerful weapon, he wrote, that the worth of a treatment is now determined not by its adoption after lengthy and serious clinical and laboratory experiments, but by the amount of advertisement it was given. It is hard not to sympathise with him.

Excess fat, he declared, was a syndrome. It had no known elementary origin, whether glandular, nervous, genital, alimentary, toxic or gastro-intestinal, but was born of complex pre-disposing causes and complex determinatives which, unfortunately, medicine had not yet been able to detect or classify. It required multiple and varied therapies, beginning with detoxication. By making selections from dietetic treatments, by judiciously employing detoxication, rest and regeneration of the assimilative functions, myotherapy (muscle therapy), opotherapy (using animal gland extracts, usually thyroid or adrenal), as well as other experimental therapies, principally electrotherapy, he believed that medicine would eventually be able to map out a definite cure and even bring with it 'the sensation of absolute physical rebirth'. Frumusan described two classes of the obese: florids and torpids, usually manifested by a 'great general enlargement of the bust, prominent abdomen, fat cheeks, double chin and fat neck, ruddy, high-coloured face (plethoric obesity), or pale and puffy (anaemic obesity)', and some instances of 'the most freakish distribution of adipose tissue'. While some very fat people had refined, 'normal' facial features, some of the 'lesser obese' had jowls, triple chins and overflowing napes. A person's weight, he calculated, should broadly equal, in kilos, the number of centimetres over a metre of the person's height.

Summing up the ways in which excess fat had been treated so far, Frumusan made a list as follows:

1. Quacks and charlatans, including those making recommendations in newspapers of products containing thyroid extract. This was dangerous claptrap.
2. Diets and thermal stations. Although a more scientific development these placed too much emphasis on the diet (and starvation) of the wealthy. In Germany and Austria, at Marienbad, Carlsbad, Kissingen, Apenta and Hamburg, the doctors attached to thermal stations were considered negligible and harmful accessories by the hotel syndicate who surrounded the patients with champagne, *thés dansants*, suppers, gaming rooms and bars. There was no tiresome discipline or anti-fats here, just a bit of bath-time galvanisation to soften and melt unwanted flesh, followed by a high colonic irrigation.
3. Medicines. Secret remedies (iodine, arsenic, alkalies, various serums, oxygen, thyroid injections) are all recommended and all fail. There was no specific medicine for obesity because it was not an illness, but a complex syndrome varying in each individual.
4. Physical agents. Heat, dry or moist in the form of vapour baths, or luminous, in the form of light-baths, such treatments were utterly useless and extremely dangerous for the majority of fat people because of the risk of heart strain. Taking a light-bath meant being submitted for half an hour to a temperature of 65 degrees centigrade, to emerge dripping with perspiration, one's heart beating to breaking point, gasping for breath, brain on fire, and then to undergo either a cold douche followed by massage or a hydroelectric iodised bath which has no effect on fat. In addition, no preliminary examinations were made before the application of such therapies.

5. Massage. Quacks, again in thermal stations, treat the fat with ointments devoid of effect. Massage has frenzied devotees and detractors but is not a cure.

6. Electricity. The hydroelectric-faradic baths administered in quack institutes 'merely serve to occupy and overawe the patients'.

7. Movement. Exercise, along with diet and medicinal treatment, gave astonishing but temporary results. Detoxication (fasting) must come first then the abdominal belt must be worn to combat overwhelming lassitude which bends the body. The belt had to be constantly adjusted; it prevented rupture and helped strengthen the abdominal wall.

8. Galvanisation and iodised ionisation. An intense galvanic current first softened then rapidly melted any fat. A four-celled hydroelectric bath with ionised compresses (vast individual electrodes whose negative poles are impregnated with a solution of iodide of sodium and bring all the regions to be treated within the sphere of an intense galvanic current) was good for 'tonification'.

9. Morphological reconstruction. This was muscular repair by galvanic current (above) plus physical exercise, but under no circumstances should it be left to over-zealous quacks.

10. Dietetics. After fasting comes correct, restricted feeding. A glass of water can be taken on waking, toast for breakfast, water between meals, grilled meat or fish for lunch, mashed potatoes, green vegetables and fruit. Dinner would be vegetable soup, vegetables, toast and fruit. Mint tea could be had at bedtime. There must be no sweets or starches, spices or condiments. One should leave the table feeling hungry – this is 'pseudo-hunger' due to vacuity of the enlarged stomach, and it would gradually disappear as the stomach regains its tonicity.

There was also, according to Frumusan, the 'problem' of race. The 'Orientals', enervated by climate, customs and a diet abounding in fats, sugar and pastry, inevitably fostered a fat population. On the other hand, the 'sober races', who lived in more bleak climates and were addicted to sport and violent exercises, prepared for well-balanced future generations, where obesity was a 'hygienic error trembling on the verge of an abyss'.

Frumusan ended his work with twenty-five case histories. One, a Mademoiselle K., was forty-seven years old, 5 ft 4 in. tall, and weighed 12 st 3 lb. She suffered from florid obesity, had a very small skeleton and presented with a double chin, enormous hips and abdomen, ptosis (a downward displacement of the abdominal organs), general fatigue, gastro-intestinal disorder and auto-intoxication. After six weeks' treatment, her weight had come down to 10 st 5 lb, without any disfigurement, and without a wrinkle in her skin. The double chin had vanished, her muscles had become firm, her strength had been regained, and her general condition was such that Mlle K. apparently felt 'barely twenty'. Her weight loss of fat was actually greater than that indicated by the scale, for a vigorous musculature had been developed, allowing her to discard the abdominal belt. This physical renascence, combined with an absolute transformation in her mentality, was admired by all her relations.

Body and mind were thus shown to work together, thought Frumusan, having recognised that many fat people suffered from melancholia and apathy. They could be helped, he said, with what he called psychic treatment, ideally conducted alongside the physical treatments to enhance their efficiency and to lift the soul of the patient to serene heights. In this way the patient would develop greater pleasure and peace as well as a 'love of some occupation [and] a physical relaxation that it is perceptible in their features', and it would all be down to an 'ingenious theory of the gymnastic of the smile'. By teaching patients to smile, Frumusan calculated that their mentality would attune itself to that expression. This was an early theory of dieting psychology, which, Frumusan predicted, would ultimately 'inspire all our efforts in the psychic re-education of the obese'.

Most doctors – Webb-Johnson, for example – used psychology in a less constructive fashion, more as a stick with which to beat their patients, it being nothing short of a 'disgrace to be fat'. The American diet book author, and one-time chair of the Public Health Committee of the California Federation of Women's Clubs in Los Angeles, Dr Lulu Hunt Peters (1873–1930), certainly thought so. Hunt Peters had become well known and well-loved for her terrifically popular syndicated newspaper columns throughout the 1920s, and then for publishing a runaway bestseller, *Dieting and Health: With Key to the Calories* (1918), said to have sold two million copies in more than fifty-five editions by 1939. A model for subsequent diet books, it was aimed and marketed primarily at women and included personal testimonials and beauty hints such as how to get rid of wrinkles. 'How anyone can want to be anything but thin is beyond my intelligence,' she told her readers, 'if there is anything comparable to the joy of taking in your clothes I have not experienced it.'

All her life Hunt Peters had battled with 'the too, too solid flesh'; she was said to weigh around 220 pounds at her heaviest and she claimed to have lost seventy pounds through following her own advice. As a child she recalled being offered consolation with the idea that she would grow out of her puppy fat and have a nice shapely body when she became a woman but, she wrote, she was a delicate slip of 165 pounds when she married. She later published the first calorie-counting book explicitly for children, *Diet for Children (and Adults) and the Kalorie Kids* (1924); astonishingly, diet books for children, such as *Maggie Goes on a Diet* (2011) by Paul Kramer are still being published today.

According to Hunt Peters, three out of four adult Americans

were disgracefully overweight. As well as being a problem wide-spread in the nation, being fat was also sinful. Slimming down, on the other hand, was an indicator of strength of mind and body: it demanded self-control, commitment and displayed self-vigilance. In fact, Hunt Peters's proclamations on dieting had a nationalistic as well as a religious fervour to them: she made an analogy between the wartime crime of hoarding food and the way in which many Americans hoarded food in their own bodies. She argued for 'Watch Your Weight Anti-Kaiser Classes' where members would be publicly weighed and fined if they had not slimmed down, with proceeds going to the Red Cross. The title of her book was modelled on a best-seller by the Christian Scientist Mary Baker Eddy, *Science and Health with Key to the Scriptures* (1891).

For the Episcopalian Hunt Peters, however, it was knowing about calories that would bring ultimate salvation, and she claimed a great deal of credit for first suggesting to the American public that counting the calories was the way to gain or lose weight. Her 'key to the calories' was an extensive list of food portions each adding up to 100 calories. It was simple, she thought: the vast majority of fat people got that way from overeating and under-exercising, more through ignorance than overindulgence or laziness (though she did acknowledge that there might be those with, perhaps, thyroid conditions who could be cured by curing their illness). Dividing the world of the overweight into those whose metabolism quickly burned fat and those whose didn't, she argued that even if you ate a single bird seed and your metabolism was slow, it would add fat to your body. 'Hereafter,' Hunt Peters instructed, 'you are going to eat calories of food. Instead of saying one slice of bread, or a piece of pie, you will say 100 calories of bread, 350 calories of pie.' On a 1,200 calorie per day diet, a dieter was allowed twelve 100-calorie units of food. Her diet system was based on an ideal weight, and the formula for measurement was to take the number of inches over 5 foot of your height, multiply that by 5.5 and add 110. This equation was meant to yield an ideal weight in pounds of a 'normal' woman. The number of calories a dieter was to consume would depend upon how far their actual weight exceeded the ideal for their height. A woman's size and shape was thus becoming shorthand for her self-worth – an ideal that we do not yet seem to have shaken off.

Calorie-counting was big news in 1920s America, but in Europe the matter was undecided. Frumusan, for one, declared calorie-counting to be an erroneous theory which risked weakening the dieter through chronic underfeeding leading to visceroptosis (prolapse of the internal organs). In theory, calorie-counting was alluring, but in practice it was absurd, he said, and only presented a temporary answer. But many believed that the better-off in America were being damaged by over-nutrition, that this was to the detriment of social progress, and that this group, and not the poor, were the most in need of missionary work. Wilbur Olin Atwater (1844–1907), the influential American agricultural chemist had argued that Americans were sloppy with their food because of overabundance and were giving themselves huge and unnecessary portions. On a trip to Germany, Atwater had been fascinated by the calorimetric work of Carl Voit and Max Rubner and, back in America in the 1890s, he produced a pamphlet for the Department of Agriculture with a standard diet and food composition tables that introduced Americans (specifically housewives) to a new way of thinking about food – about proteins, carbohydrates and fats. The pamphlet began the popularisation of the concept of calories, something that scientists such as Edward Frankland (1825–99), in the study of the energy values of different foods, had been working on for some time.

Atwater and a physicist colleague built the Atwater-Rosa calorimeter, a machine to calculate the metabolic rate of, and heat produced by, test subjects undertaking various physical activities, in order to measure the balance between food intake and energy output. Their objective was not only to research energy and metabolism, but to improve dietary standards for the working classes. Atwater's work gained momentum over the following years and became ever more popular with the public – magazines such as the *Ladies' Home Journal* hired nutritionists to write regular columns on scientific feeding and eating – but it also had practical and political implications for the nation. Atwater had raised awareness of food calories, recommended a cheap and efficient diet of proteins, beans and vegetables, and fewer carbohydrates, and had made calorie-counting central to the fields of nutrition and dietetics as well as the lives of millions of dieters.

Dr Clarence Lieb of Boston advocated a calorie-controlled diet but was sufficiently old-fashioned to use it to 'engender the fear of fat' in his patients. He believed excess fat was a disease and, though he wanted to debunk diet faddism, thought that 'the fat lady who loves to eat has also an abundant mass of credulity and is ready to try anything once'. Books such as Lieb's *Eat, Drink and be Slender: What Every Overweight Person Should Know and Do* (1929), complete with the new menus and tables of 100 calorie portions, were still competing in a marketplace that included diet 'experts' of all shades and qualifications. Every variety of quack and charlatan continued to make income out of those who could pinch an inch or more and didn't much like it. The same old fat 'cures', such as rubber garments and chin-bands, were still being peddled even if their only practical effect was to hold in perspiration and allow the skin to become macerated – nothing at all like the alluring Before-and-After photographs.

Fat cures contained either desiccated thyroid, which was dangerous, or elements that were either ineffective or poisonous. Dr Lewellys F. Barker, writing on how glands affected weight, believed that the use of slimming drugs was a worrying development, 'a short cut, not to beauty but to the grave'. Some of these pills were barred from the US Mail but they were still available at local drug stores, and government scientists tasked with analysing 'fat-dissolving' preparations found five cents' worth of soft soap selling for as much as $1.50. The Postmaster General could debar fraudulent products from the post (something recorded only twice) and the Department of Agriculture could act on dubious claims on packets, but if claims were only advertised in newspapers or circulars then Federal Law was helpless.

Products came with fancy names and fancy prices: Every Woman's Flesh Reducer, Lesser Slim-Figure-Bath, Florazona ($20,000 annual sales), Fayro Bath Salts (1.5 million packets sold by 1931), Slenmar Reducing Brush, and La-mar Reducing Soap (200 to 300 orders daily). The overweight were instructed to mix powders and salts into their hot bathwater and then lie in it for ten minutes each night before bed (the only possible resultant weight loss could come from sweating). Chewing gums, such as Silph Chewing Gum, Slends Fat Reducing Chewing Gum and Elfin Fat Reducing Gum Drops often had laxatives in them, or thyroid extract, or pokeroot. Diet foods and drinks were everywhere – 'Squirt' was an early, tastefully named diet drink, apparently for 'grown-up tastes' – and by the 1980s these included Carnation 'Slender', marketed by Nestlé, controversial supplier of baby formula across the world. All these diet drinks and foods were – are – infantilising mush for grown men and women.

And there were spurious 'Reducing' breads, whole-wheat and gluten with added laxatives such as castor oil. In *The Conquest of Constipation* (1923), William S. Walsh calculated that $50,000,000 was being spent each year on laxatives. Moderation was the best temperance, he counselled, temperance is the best diet, and diet is the best doctor. One could, sighed Cramp, author of 'Fooling the Fat', but 'stand aghast at the preposterous foolishness of it all'.

Paying for and swallowing weight-loss pills and potions

might have seemed foolish but surgery to excise fat was a more worrying development, though many people remain willing to submit to both. In the 1920s, so-called beauty surgeons belonged to the 'underworld of medicine', according to Dr Joseph Colt Bloodgood (1867–1935), a respected cancer pathologist. His work on the 'Possibilities and Dangers of Beauty Operations, and the Dangers of Excessive Fat in Surgery and Disease' praised the discipline of plastic surgery, which had developed in the aftermath of the First World War, but considered this a different beast to beautification by the knife, something that was treated with suspicion and derided in the 'best circles of the profession'. Beauty surgery was really a very small part of the wider field of plastic surgery, and only justified if 'deformity is very pronounced' (though Bloodgood doesn't say how, or by whom, a deformity is identified, or, indeed, who judges whether it is ugly or not).

Beauty surgeons, he sniffed, worked strictly on a commercial basis. Methods of local anaesthesia were easy to master and demands for surgery meant it was increasingly lucrative. These surgeons recognised a group of people who were nothing less than deluded, according to Bloodgood, and who were 'willing to suffer pain and prolonged discomfort, and to spend the last of their own money, or money obtained from others, in the cost of treatment'. People with what he called visible defects which destroy their beauty and symmetry – scars, double chins due to fat, breasts that are too large or too small, pendulous, heavy fat hanging from the abdomen, fat about the feet and ankles – were willing to pay fees out of all proportion to the character of the work done. They had a 'mental twist' which made them 'easy prey to any dishonest individual, in or out of the medical profession'. Beauty doctors preyed on these women, made a good living out of them, and should be exposed. Their patients were only satisfied for a short time and then their *idée fixe* returned, they became dissatisfied with the correction or another supposed deformity that needed correcting. This demand, and the unscrupulous beauty experts who furnished the supply, was a problem for the medical profession, and it was up to doctors to provide a corrective: 'The great danger to individuals who seek the advice of such beauty surgeons is that they will get an operation or a treatment whether it is indicated or not.' This, remember, is the 1920s, yet we are still having the same debate today.

If the removal of fat by the knife was deemed necessary, then only the best doctor should be consulted – money obviously counted – and before any operation was performed the patient should undergo a systematic general reduction by diet, exercise and massage. Fat was already known to be a risk under anaesthetic, and wounds in very fat people were considered more apt to break down and suppurate. There was a danger of fat necrosis in which, due to faulty circulation, fat would liquify like an emulsion and, ten to fifteen days after a procedure, could burst through a skin wound. Bloodgood warned against the removal of fat from double or triple chins which hang between the neck and thyroid gland because this sort of operation would neither improve looks nor make them worse, and the fat would in any case rapidly reform; there was the added possibility of multiple lipomas (tumours composed of fat). Surgery carried a risk of scarring, which he considered very ugly, and which by no means always responded to treatment by x-rays and radium. While he recognised the difficult problem of 'fat armpits in modern evening dresses', he didn't think surgery was the way to go. He had, after all, seen more than 5,000 pairs of breasts in thirty years and could only recommend dieting to reduce them. If he was asked to operate he said, 'My answer is: Emphatically, no: with rare exceptions.'

But some fat did require surgery, according to Bloodgood's colleague, Dr Howard A. Kelly (1858–1943), first Professor of Gynaecology at Johns Hopkins Hospital, Baltimore. No dressmaker or corset could 'neutralize the deformity of a pendulous abdomen' of an extreme degree. Kelly was possibly the first to perform an abdominal apronectomy, the removal of an apron of fat in 'huge elliptical pieces' from the bellies of obese women who had to be operated on for other reasons, such as hernias. In 1899 he had removed a pendulous abdomen weighing 14.9 pounds from a 285-pound woman (three years earlier another doctor had removed twenty-five pounds of fat from the same woman's breasts). Kelly often cut away up to twenty, thirty, even fifty pounds, of skin and fat from his female patients. These women would, in pursuit of a fast result (and he, presumably, of a fast buck), suffer risk, pain and prolonged discomfort, not to mention the exorbitant costs. Even though he made sure that any physical scar, 'however unsightly', was never seen, Kelly did admit that the operations usually failed in the long term because patients did not go on to diet and exercise.

It seemed strange to Bloodgood that doctors had been preaching for twenty years or so on cancer and tuberculosis, but that in 1920s America there was no society for the prevention and control of obesity among the populace. In this period, a patronising tone was inherent in the way doctors approached their patients, fat or otherwise. Dr Frank Evans of Pittsburgh, a pioneer of the very low calorie diet, thought that, though many people sincerely believed that they weren't large eaters and 'mention with hope and longing some gland trouble', they should be reminded that fat is a 'tangible material, and that there is no gland with an aperture through which it can be introduced, [it] is not rubbed through the skin, does not enter the eyes as views, nor through the ears as sound'. Glands could not make something out of nothing and people could not be relied upon to take responsibility for themselves.

The early thirties in America were, of course, the time of the Great Depression and the medical profession showed more and more interest in the American diet in the midst of economic crisis, unemployment, poverty and hunger marches. The same was true for interwar Britain. While the wealthier bought up slimming foods, books and aids, the diet of the poor was severely constrained. Neither were the upper classes perceived as being particularly prone to obesity; rather this was a problem that beset the more sedentary and increasingly affluent middle classes. Leonard Williams, in *Obesity*, had looked to heredity and social change to explain it, comparing the leaner, taller aristocracy 'whose ancestors through the ages have had no necessity for hoarding fat' with 'the profiteer, and the nouveau-riche ... always depicted as bull-necked and pot-bellied – which he generally is'. Williams's stereotyping didn't end there. Just as Craston had argued in the 1890s, Williams laid a large part of the blame for the fat of the middle-class male on wives who, he thought, overfed their husbands so that they would be easy-going, yielding, uncritical and stupid. The rot began when husbands were in their thirties and by the time they reached fifty 'the sinister process is in full swing'. The obesity expert W. F. Christie also targeted 'well-to-do' married middle-class women. He found gender differences in his analysis of medical histories of 184 fat people, 75 per cent of whom were female. 'Surplus fat,' he wrote, 'should neither be tolerated with resignation, nor left for concealment to the tailoring craft.' It was the 'obvious duty of every member of a civilized community' to lose weight and rid themselves of the social unhappiness, physical inefficiency and shorter lifespan which excessive fat entailed. Fat, according to Williams, was a 'malignant and merciless parasite', it was disgusting, pathological and degenerate, and was due to self-indulgence and greed – so it was quite common among criminals, embezzlers and homosexuals.

But the new female fashion of thinness was also undoubtedly a bad – and sexually perverse – thing as it was not achieved in order to attract 'normal, red-blooded men' but was a 'ruse to find favour in the eyes of the degenerates and homosexuals'.

Moderation in one's eating habits was the way to live a good and a long life. If you dieted too much you became deviant and if you overindulged it would lead to an early death because, as Christie bluntly put it, 'More people floated into their coffins on a flood of beef tea and milk than ever arrive there by the ravages of disease.' This is the same complaint made in the sixteenth century about more people dying from overeating than ever had by the sword or plague. Just as today, there were anxieties about the consequences of over-civilised, modern, urban living.

The culprits, then, were middle-aged men and their greed, women and their vanity, and the degenerate poor, who were guilty of general ignorance. Moral condemnation seeped through all this, suggesting that those who were fat and inactive were failing their country and the empire. Sir George Newman (1870–1948), Chief Medical Officer of the newly established Ministry of Health, had stressed ignorance and lack of self-control rather than poverty as causal factors in the poor physical condition of the lower classes who were wanted to fight in the Great War (this despite it being commonly known that a working-class woman would sacrifice her own meals to feed her family and bread-winner). Newman believed that public health reform rested on the reform of an individual's personal life, on moderation, cleanliness and good habits, and that this was every man's first contribution to the State and a 'primary asset of the British Empire'. In 1926 he attacked excessive and unsuitable food and a lack of fresh air and exercise as sowing the dangerous seeds of national degeneration. He did accept, in 1931, that some were going hungry but continued to argue that many were 'over-fed – giving their bodies little rest, clogging them with yet more food'. Health, he wrote, could only be achieved by the people themselves, 'a nation becomes physically strong and healthy if each individual so cultivates his own body and mind as to live at the top of his physical, mental and moral capacity. This means an ordered way of life ... every adult must discipline and train himself, or be trained ... to understand and practise this art of Living – much of the essence of which is contained in the Greek aphorism, "know thyself and be moderate in all things".'

These anxieties ran parallel to an emerging physical culture of personal discipline, dieting and exercise that included sunbathing and changes in fashion for men and women which brought greater freedom of dress. Images of beautiful, fit bodies accompanied the growing interest in the eugenics movement and a resurgence of fears about racial deterioration. The public were lectured to and encouraged in their hygienic habits, self-control, personal responsibility and civic duty. New societies and pressure groups, such as Sir William Arbuthnot Lane's New Health Society, were launched during the 1920s. Members included Leonard Williams and Frederick Hornibrook (1877–1936), author of the best-selling *The Culture of the Abdomen: The Cure of Obesity and Constipation* (1933), and Hornibrook's wife, Ettie Rout, whose own book, *Sex and Exercise: A study of the Sex Function in Women and its Relation to Exercise* (1925) was aimed specifically at women. Hornibrook dealt in the maintenance of the ideal body, a popular homage to the Greek aesthetic. There was never, he said, one solitary instance of beauty 'fashioned in fatness'. He, too, was disgusted by the all too common sight of 'fat, ugly, clumsy bodies', and he pitied those with protuberant bellies, ponderous buttocks, and 'their cumbrous waddle through life'. His *Culture of the Abdomen*, widely recommended by the medical profession, made no mention of calories but espoused a system of seven minutes' daily abdominal exercises based on Maori dances, and a regular retraction of the abdominal muscles throughout the day. Thorough mastication was encouraged, plus drinking lots of water, moderate eating, and 'activating the bowel'.

Ettie Rout had adapted the system for women, making a

direct link between the health of the digestive organs and a good reproductive function. *Sex and Exercise*, republished in 1934 as *Stand Up and Slim Down: Being Restoration Exercises for Women with a Chapter on Food Selection in Constipation and Obesity*, claimed that abdominal, pelvic and hip exercises combined with a high-fibre diet were essential to getting a slim, beautiful figure. These practices also enhanced efficiency in sexual inter-course, pregnancy and labour – women were, after all, the 'race mothers'. This 'Racial Health' was widely promoted elsewhere too, by the likes of the Women's League of Health and Beauty, a famous physical culture organisation launched in 1930.

A healthy, efficient female physique accompanied the changes in fashion and the rise in beauty culture. The ideal female body was now less voluptuous, more straight-waisted, with well-developed muscles and broad hips. Ettie, wrote her husband, was the only woman he had ever met who came up to this Venus de Milo standard. Sturdiness and strength were the important factors, and he condemned the diet fads for risking the physical health of women and turning them into nervous wrecks like the semi-invalid and ultra-feminine finicky eaters of the previous century. Excessive dieting, he argued, not only resulted in ill-health, but also in an inevitable loss of beauty; it made women thin and scraggy with an 'aged, deeply-lined and discontented appearance' which even 'liberal make-up will not successfully hide'. The *British Medical Journal* fretted that 'the sex which for many years injured its health by tight-lacing is not likely to be deterred from slimming by such considerations. The dictates of fashion will be paramount.'

Expectations of and for women had been changing since the war and were reflected in fashion, beauty products and advertis-ing. But fear and opposition to such changes was also prevalent and anxieties about the female role and what constituted the feminine constantly surfaced. This conflict wasn't played out only in popular culture – science was also struggling with the idea of femininity and producing drugs and synthetic hormones which shaped bodies and behaviours. Film, radio, newspapers, magazines and billboards proliferated during this period and gave out mixed messages to men and women alike, all against the prevailing undercurrent of anxiety about the sins of greed and pride. Through the workings of politics, publicity, science and vanity the Western world was definitely in the grip of the new 'slimming craze'.

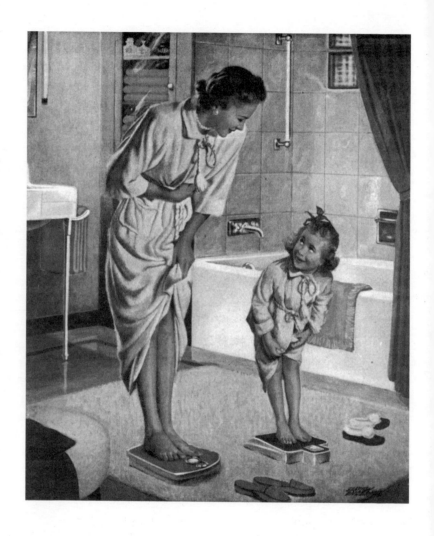

8. In the 1870s weighing scale companies began producing their machines for people as well as for foods and produce. The first public penny-scales began to appear on railway stations, in shops and restaurants, hotels, cinemas, banks and office buildings and started bringing in the millions. In the beginning they played you a tune, read your fortune and could even 'Speak Your Weight', though they soon became silent. Bathroom scales arrived soon after the First World War making dieting something that could be measured from home and the mother's dieting history became her daughter's dieting future.

8

Half a Grapefruit and Two Olives

BY THE 1930S, dieting was everywhere. In 1931, Francis G. Benedict, Director of the Carnegie Institute's Nutrition Laboratory, remarked that 'the interest in weight reduction is so great that the lecturer on physiology, medicine or nutrition has but to introduce the words "weight reduction" at any part of his discourse to change a quiet, sleepy group into an eager, agitated, expectant band of zealots'. In that year, too, the character actor Louis Wollheim collapsed and died after losing twenty-five pounds in a month, trying to keep his part in the film, *The Front Page*. Paul Whiteman, the most popular bandleader in America (Duke Ellington called him the 'King of Jazz'), lost 113 pounds in a year in order to woo his fourth and last wife, and published *Whiteman's Burden* in 1933, dedicated to 'the 24,000,000 fat people in the world generally'. In England, the same year, the *Lancet* was telling its readers that there was 'no more popular subject of discussion among the laity than the reduction of weight'. The popular American nutritionist Victor Lindlahr held a radio 'reducing party' in 1936 and 26,000 people nationwide joined up to his idea. His diet book, *You Are What You Eat* (1942), went on to sell nearly a million copies and just one of his radio broadcasts on dieting could attract up to 35,000 letters. Everyone was thinking or worrying about being fat and everyone was going on a diet.

Civilisation was definitely to blame. So wrote Dr Ernest E. Claxton in *Weight Reduction: Diet and Dishes, with Recipes by Lucy Burdekin* (1937), and he received a glowing review in the *Lancet* for adhering to the ancient notion of a causal relationship between fat and decadence. The switch from hunting to housing was the prehistoric start of the problem, he asserted with absolutely no evidence, and the noble savage was never, ever, fat: 'Hundreds of generations and thousands of years had passed and had brought with them a change in man's physique.' Harnessing a convenient quasi-evolutionary theory, Claxton deduced that some of our organs had atrophied and some of our glands had deteriorated, and that this process had combined with the increased activity of our brains and other parts of the body to meet our new requirements. The fat man, heredity his curse, was the result of this process, and he could not help but 'excite the interest and comment of his more fortunate brothers', like some sort of freakish missing link.

Claxton's programme was a progressive prophylactic one designed to educate, but some of the accompanying assumptions were decidedly unscientific. Calories, or food value, were understood as the amount of energy a food provided, and dieters were advised to eat normal quantities at mealtimes but to make sure everything was of low calorie content. You could only lose weight by taking food that is lower in value than the body's energy requirements. Claxton was anxious to point out that no 'slimming diet' need entail severe restrictions, be unbearably monotonous or sickeningly unpalatable. What absolutely did have to be borne in mind, however, was that 'the secret of success is to be found in the willingness of the subject to submit himself to a disciplined diet. Short cuts are no good.' Perseverance in your course of action, secrecy, will-power, submission and discipline were the necessary virtues of successful dieting. Creatively quoting St Paul – 'Let us lay aside every weight … lay aside the sin that doth so easily beset us' – Claxton interpreted this as a lecture against gluttony and fat. The problem may easily beset us but it was not going to be so easy to rectify it – dieters could be forgiven for feeling defeated before they even began.

The drawbacks of being fat were legion, wrote Claxton, but the worst was that being big meant being a butt for humour. Distinguishing himself from some earlier, more crude commentators, he asked, 'why do we laugh or want to laugh at the fat man?' The fat were now the one exception that people were allowed to laugh at because of their 'deformity' where once 'the dwarf, the giant, the hunchback, the cripple, the thin man, the fat man, and so on' were all considered a great joke. But Claxton couldn't, unfortunately, quite bring himself to deny the joke; one 'must still admit, however, that a fat man or woman looks funny'. Perhaps, he speculated, it was a lack of proportion in the fat body; perhaps the set of the mouth and eyes and the folds of the face are similar to the expression associated with laughter and so everyone laughs 'with' the fat person. But he thought it more likely that it was an intrinsic lack of dignity in a fat body, a mild ungainliness which 'tickles us'. The fat man is often a funny man, he mused, but 'is he funny because he is fat or fat because he is funny?' The mental and physical make-up of the individual, argued Claxton, 'depended much upon his glandular outfit, efficiency or inefficiency, and the humorous vein of many certainly goes with some degree of obesity … it is a distinct disadvantage to be fat, for they can rarely be taken seriously'.

Claxton wasn't alone in these musings. In America, Dr Morris Fishbein thought that temperament was an important factor in actually causing weight gain and that the assumption that fat people were easy-going was probably quite wrong. Up to 60 per cent of people who are overweight claimed, he reported, to be of an excitable and nervous disposition and only 10 per cent were phlegmatic. Just think about it, he suggested, encouraging his readers in their prejudices, 'if you happen to know an excitable fat person, you will realise that such a person appears to be much more excitable than an excitable thin person … temperament is not important in reduction of weight, but it is important from the point of view of the will power of the person concerned in following a strictly scientific reducing diet'.

It had often been remarked, wrote Claxton, that the civilised races dig their graves with their teeth. Everyone, Claxton reminded his readers, should remember that fat must come from somewhere: 'If it does not come from food,' he asked, 'where does it come from?' People had to understand the correlation between intake and output. Some fat people consistently overate, as notions of fatness and ideas of normal portions varied so greatly. Others were inclined to panic and drink large quantities of cold water, or take violent exercise, thus doing themselves more harm than good and making them feel more tired and hungry, thereby increasing their appetites and so their size. Not only did society abhor the fat person but the dictates of fashion did, too, and another popular reason for slimming, he conjectured, was that 'not only is the fat man hard on his clothing, but also hard on the furniture'. Fat was costly in so many ways, he continued: take the 'difficulty of finding room in an overcrowded vehicle [which] has to be experienced to be appreciated'. And life insurance was hard to get, too. Some overweight citizens would always be prevailed upon through extravagantly worded advertisements in their newspapers to try some patent drug or restrict their food intake and make themselves dangerously ill. Claxton especially warned his readers against thyroid medications, telling them always to consult their doctor. They should have a sugar lump if they felt faint and must avoid constipation by eating plenty of fruit and vegetables, and swallowing the odd dose of liquid paraffin.

He particularly recommended the milk and banana diet, a simple reducing regimen designed by the American physician, Dr Harrop. Bananas and skimmed milk were the main items of nourishment and the idea was to alternate these with one or two restricted meals or to eat just them, by themselves, for a week to ten days. One could have six large, ripe bananas with four glasses of skimmed milk a day, making 768 calories, with perhaps some other low calorie foods, for example, clear soup, bran biscuits, lettuce or green vegetables. He helpfully noted that, 'for those who dislike bananas this method can have no application'.

For whichever diet one chose, Claxton laid down nine 'General Rules for Weight Reduction':

1. Ascertain the calorie requirements for the desired weight. One's type of work or daily output of energy must come into this calculation.
2. Decide upon the method of dieting which is to be adopted. The choice may be made from the following five options:
   a. Starvation diet.
   b. Basal diet – where minimum food to support life at rest is taken.
   c. Maintenance diet – taking sufficient food to provide energy for the desired weight.
   d. Decreasing to maintenance diet – a diet that provides sufficient energy to support the present weight; this is gradually reduced to the level of the maintenance diet.
   e. Qualitative restriction – a diet for milder cases: fats, sugar and excess carbohydrates are avoided.

3. Persevere in the prescribed diet. This must be carried out with consistency. Sugar, sweets and alcohol in all forms, if taken, must be included only within the limits of the total daily calorie allowance, but it is best to avoid them altogether.

4. Avoid salt, sauces and condiments that increase the appetite.

5. Take plenty of exercise. Brisk walking, golf, tennis, rowing, physical exercises, and so on, may be enjoyed, but be careful not to undo the good that the increase of exercise will do by taking more food than is prescribed.

6. Avoid long nights in bed (if the doctor allows this).

7. Take a cold bath daily (if the doctor allows this).

8. Masticate well, and the smaller meals will be more satisfying.

9. Watch the weight. Care must be taken that the treatment is not overdone.

Some circumstances could not help, he admitted, but work against the fat person: age, illness, alcohol, living in the tropics, menopause and gland problems, all potentially made losing weight much more difficult, and women were more afflicted by excess fat than men. Glands, their functions and extracts, had been, as we have seen, the subject of enthusiastic scientific research in the late nineteenth century and had become big news in the first decades of the twentieth, peddled to the public as elixirs of life. Consequently, they cropped up in most diet books as body-enhancers. Mrs C. F. Leyel's offering, *Diet and Commonsense* (1936), regarded glandular problems as the source of weight troubles, and medication as a cure. 'To be too fat is not only uncomfortable,' she wrote, 'it is unhealthy, because it means that the glands are not functioning properly, or that there is a lack of iron or sodium.' Thanks to modern science she could tell her readers that there was now no need for such a condition, and that it was no longer regarded as a necessary evil of middle life. People who remained thin all through life were usually those who had an over-active thyroid or pituitary gland, or both, and now these glands could be encouraged and increased by extracts or glands taken medicinally and by special dieting.

Mrs Leyel (1880–1957) didn't say whether she had taken glandular extracts but she had successfully used the controversial Hollywood Diet Sheet as a way to get thin, and she included it in her book. The eighteen-day plan was tantamount to near starvation. The first three days, for example, went like this:

First Day
Breakfast: One half grapefruit. One egg. One slice Melba toast.
Lunch : Six slices cucumber. Tea or coffee.
Dinner: Two eggs. One half of lettuce. One tomato. One
    half grapefruit.

Second Day
Breakfast: One orange. One egg. One slice Melba toast.
Lunch : Lettuce. Tea.
Dinner: Grilled steak (plain). One tomato. One half
    lettuce. One half grapefruit. Tea or coffee.

Third Day
Breakfast: One half grapefruit. Six slices cucumber.
Lunch: One egg. Lettuce. Tea or coffee.
Dinner: One lamb chop (trim fat before cooking). One
    egg. Three radishes, two olives. One half grapefruit.
    Lettuce. Tea or coffee.

And by the time you got to Day Eighteen it was no better, and possibly worse, consisting of just one egg, two tomatoes, half a grapefruit and coffee, and, at dinner, one grilled fish, the other half of your grapefruit, more coffee and some plain spinach.

Rose M. Simmonds, a State Registered Nurse and Dietician at the Hammersmith and London Hospitals, had a slightly more scientific approach. In her *Handbook of Diets* (1931) she emphasised that, having ascertained the standard weight for the dieter, one should measure their height, find out their age and consult tables. The diet should then be arranged to include at at least three ounces of protein for every stone of the standard body weight, and then one could make up the required number of calories with the carbohydrates and fat foods. On this diet she thought it possible that an overweight person might lose between 2 and 6 stone in two months. One could have more fruit and green salad if still hungry, but absolutely no sugar, fried or starchy foods, as the large couldn't have these without putting on considerable amounts of weight. Bread and potatoes could be gradually included as one's weight approached normal levels. She offered some consolation by saying that most people who gave up sugar for a good while would lose their desire for sweet foods. And, in opposition to Claxton, she banned bananas outright. Her reducing diet is as follows:

Breakfast
Tea, milk, 5 tablespoons
2 eggs, or a piece of fish, or 1 thin rasher of bacon
1 'Vita Weat' biscuit
Butter, piece size of half a walnut
Tomatoes, quarter lb fresh, or any kind of fresh fruit

Dinner
Lean meat or cheese – a good portion (about 3 oz)
A good plateful of green vegetables or salad
1 small apple, orange, pear or grapefruit
1 'Vita Weat' biscuit

Tea
Tea, milk, 5 tablespoons
1 egg
1 'Vita Weat' biscuit
Butter, piece size of half a walnut

Supper
Steamed fish, a fair portion (about 6 oz), or lean meat and
    cheese
Butter, piece size of two walnuts
A good plateful of green vegetables or salad
1 small apple, orange, pear or grapefruit
1 'Vita Weat' biscuit

This made a daily total of approximately 1,168 calories. Her
reducing diet for growing children has more protein and approximately 1,342 calories. Most overweight people, she argued,
simply eat too much and, in particular, too much carbohydrate.
And, in her experience, they often told her that they had only
very small appetites, that they never ate a good meal, and so
on. But on questioning her patients she could generally elicit
information such as that the dieter always tasted the food when
cooking, thereby taking in many excess calories throughout the
day, that he or she was overly fond of sweetstuff, or ate a lot of
bread and potatoes.

To illustrate this problem Miss Simmonds recalled that a
young woman, aged twenty-five, weighing 14 stone, had arrived
at the London Hospital outpatient dietary department, having
failed to respond to dietary treatments that included thyroid.
It turned out that though she had strictly followed her doctor's orders, she had kept to her long-standing habit of eating a
pound of chocolates every day. She was persuaded to stop eating
chocolates, and lost 3 stone in six months. Another successful

case was that of a boy, aged sixteen, weighing 21 stone, who was sent into the metabolism ward for weight reduction. This boy had been in hospital several times before but had never lost weight, until they discovered that he was continually eating acid drops, up to a pound of them, daily. He was kept in the metabolism ward for six weeks in order to break him of the habit, and on discharge he weighed 17 stone 10 lb, having lost 4 stone since admission. His hospital diet was composed of 2 ounces of carbohydrates, 3 ounces of protein and 2 ounces of fat. After nine months his weight had fallen to 11 stone 2 lb. Doctors then increased his intake by adding a pint of milk daily and bread in small amounts. After two years the boy was able to eat a normal diet without gaining weight, though he always had to limit his consumption of sugar. During the whole of this period, Miss Simmonds recorded, he was given no drugs and took only gentle exercise.

At the other extreme, discussing diet in anorexia, she noted that the patient, 'for various reasons will not eat the food given him, even in small amounts'. At the London Hospital all food was given in liquid form (with the exception of rusks) and 'a feed is given every two hours [and] sometimes the patient is awakened for the necessary night feeds', which sounds very much like a baby's regimen. This may have had a psychologically infantilising effect, as personal responsibility was surrendered: a nurse was instructed to stand by the patient while the food, which was given in very small amounts, was consumed so that doctors would know exactly how much the patient had had; no opportunity was given for the anorexic to dispose of it in any way other than by drinking it.

The medical viewpoint in the 1930s was that what constituted excess fat was difficult to define and highly personal until, of course, it became obvious that one's health was being damaged. Professor Charles Lambie (1891–1961) of the University of

Sydney, writing in the *British Medical Journal* (1935), thought that the aesthetic criterion of fat was too often determined by individual taste or the 'dictates of fashion'. He was anxious to claim obesity for the medical profession by explaining that there came a point at which the deposition of fat would impair a person's functional activity and give rise to symptoms. So someone may be said to be too fat if their adiposity resulted in distress or discomfort of any kind, impaired the sense of well-being, or diminished the capacity to enjoy life. The physician, he made clear, was called upon to regard excess fat as a disfigurement, as a disease or as a 'sign'. Ultimately, by 'embarrassing' the heart and respiration and diminishing the resistance to disease it could turn out to be a menace to life itself. Even where it did not introduce any deleterious results, obesity could be a feature of various disorders, some of which could shorten life, as shown by the life expectancy data of insurance companies. But these tables were constructed as a standard of normality rather than a criterion of disease, and taking people at random was, he said, not really a good measurement. People would appear less abnormal if they were selected according to their build, that the 'correct' weight for an individual should in some degree be related to his or her physical type. Lambie wanted, rightly, to emphasise that if this were more widely realised 'many people would avoid ill-health and privation through ill-advised attempts to make their bodily configuration conform to some general standard, whether derived from ideal weight formulae or prescribed by fashion'.

Professor Lambie's paper, 'Obesity: Aetiology and Metabolism', was an important forerunner of many such studies in the decades since. Fat, he wrote, was first broken down in the intestine into fatty acids, which formed soaps and glycerol, but in the process of absorption through the intestinal wall these were again synthesised into fat. Carbohydrate was probably the main source of body fat, accounting for about two-thirds of the energy of an ordinary mixed diet, though he thought that protein might also cause fat in some circumstances. It was all to do with taking in more energy than you required – the excess foodstuff had to be stored, chiefly in the form of fat. It was reasonable to suppose that obesity would result whenever there was long-continued excess of intake over output of energy, thus disturbing the energy balance. Disturbances to basal metabolic rate (the amount of energy consumed while the body is at rest) might include drugs, such as thyroid or dinitrophenol, the toxins of disease, and one's emotional state, especially a tendency to worry, though he didn't agree with the assumption that ageing meant getting fatter. Lambie did think obesity was more common among people with sluggish habits and sedentary occupations, and many of his patients dated their obesity from a period of enforced rest, such as an illness or pregnancy – the greater incidence of obesity in women could, he deduced, be attributable to these factors. But often the sluggishness was actually a late effect of obesity, when movement was diminished.

Altogether it was easier for fat people to lose weight by reducing their food intake than by increasing their exercise (and too much exercise might stimulate appetite as well as lead to injury). It was obvious to Lambie that there were also people who were big eaters and who, in spite of a sedentary lifestyle, failed to increase in weight, while others who took a fraction of the amount of food and lead a more active life became ever fatter. This suggested that the problem of obesity was complicated and not simply a question of adjusting one's requirements. Water retention (possibly a lack of thyroid secretion), lowered metabolism, or a discrepancy between estimated and actual energy requirements might all be factors. Though the body could deal with excess caloric intake by limiting absorption, elimination, increased activity or combustion, it was usually a case of excess consumption and storage, or 'luxus'. (Some seventy years later, in 2006, an article in *Agriculture and Human Values* redefined the term 'luxus consumption' to mean food waste as well as over-consumption and storage of body fat. In other words, overeating is understood today as a social phenomenon with serious environmental, as well as personal, costs and consequences.

Lambie thought that most people were prone to overeat, taking food in excess of their energy requirements, though in most cases this was effectively dealt with by the body's natural weight regulation, lowering and increasing the rate of metabolism. The average intake of food per head of population in 1935 was approximately 3,400 calories (according to Atwater), and the average physiological requirement was only 2,500 to 3,000 calories, leaving an excess of 400 to 900 calories per head. Yet only a small proportion of the population was obese. Variations in luxus consumption would explain these differences. There was no evidence, he maintained, that the obese were bad at burning fat, that the liver, which is supposed to convert fat into a form suitable for oxidation, was at fault, nor that there was any particular problem in burning carbohydrate, so luxus consumption and increased storage were the most likely culprits.

In 1937 Dr Fishbein published his second popular diet book in London and New York, this one called *Your Diet and Your Health*. It was dedicated to his wife, Anna, 'whose culinary accomplishments in the younger years of my married life and whose graduate studies in this field in later years have maintained a constant war between my weight and my appetite'. Most diet-book writers, such as Cornaro, Cheyne and Banting, had had their own weight problems to work through and some were more evangelical than others in their desire to shock the fat and spread the weight-loss word.

Over a lifetime of three score years and ten, wrote Fishbein, a human being consumes 1,400 times his body weight. This equates to over 200,000 pounds of material and includes 6,000 loaves of bread, 3 oxen, 4 calves, 8 hogs, 4 sheep, 300 chickens, 75 geese and 100 pigeons (if he did not eat pigeons he made up for it with something else), 2,000 large fish, 3,000 sardines, flounders and herring. He would also eat about 9,000 pounds of potatoes, 12,000 pounds of other vegetables, 14,000 pounds of fruit and 6,000 quarts (9,992 UK pints) of milk. If he was German, Fishbein thought he would most likely also include 15,000 quarts (24,980 UK pints) of beer. He would take in up to 12,000 quarts (19,984 UK pints) of coffee, 1,000 pounds of salt, 5,000 eggs, 8,000 pounds of sugar, 2,000 pounds of cheese, 10,000 quarts (16,653 UK pints) of water, and 'a lot of smaller delicacies'. This gargantuan list of mixed foods puts one in mind of Gillian McKeith's tasteless television programme *You Are What You Eat* with its rather foul spreads of her fat victim's weekly intake. It must have been designed to have a similar effect: to sicken the potential dieter.

Fishbein again pulled no punches. A man doing hard work would, he estimated, burn up about 4,150 calories a day, a moderate worker would use 3,400 calories, a desk worker required 2,700 calories, and ladies of leisure who slept late in the morning and who played bridge or attended a matinee in the afternoon and did not dance too long at night would need only 2,450 calories. And that was why ladies of leisure who read the tabloids and munched chocolates enhanced their avoirdupois until they got way beyond being what he called pleasantly plump. Not only that, but such women would soon find that 'rolls of fat accumulate in places from which they ought to be absent and lines of worry appear on their foreheads'. All those chocolates were changed into fat and stored in the body.

The daily requirement for sugar was around twelve to eighteen ounces. No one had yet determined the minimum amount of sugar that a person required, but it was generally believed that one shouldn't have less than about three and a half ounces of sugar per day for any length of time. The average American had a pretty sweet tooth, Fishbein thought, and there had been a gradual rise in the consumption of sugars from 15 pounds per year in 1825, to 60 pounds in 1900, and 115 pounds in 1925. When Fishbein published *Your Diet and Your Health* in 1937 the figure was back to 100 pounds, 'but that is still much more sugar proportionately than is eaten by any other nation in the world'. Dr Mary Swartz Rose (1874–1941), Professor of Nutrition and ardent educator of the public (in the Great War she devised scientific, balanced diets for the American army and helped develop army rations), had said that sugar creates an appetite not for other foods but for itself, and so should be treated with caution. Older people tending towards fat, and who should be careful about overeating, should avoid excessive amounts of sugars and starches. He or she was advised to avoid cereals, potatoes, macaroni and spaghetti, except in small quantities, and everyone, at fifty-five years of age, should eat and drink a little less each year.

A generally accepted truism was that the way to prevent excess weight gain was to cultivate sufficient willpower and avoid eating too much food, and, to this end, there was one exercise that was of the greatest importance: 'It involves turning the head slowly from left to right and back again, in the gesture that means "no", when food is passed.' Still, it was not as easy as that, obviously, and investigations indicated that the discipline required to maintain a reduction in weight was too severe for most of those who weighed too much. It had frequently been found that the parents of overweight people were themselves inclined to be overweight, and that bad eating habits had been passed on. The truism that fat could be learned is still accepted today.

In the late 1930s, Fishbein was recommending a diet of 1,200 calories a day (providing the necessary proteins, carbohydrates, fats, mineral salts and vitamins) but, despite this, and without recognising that he might in fact be part of the problem, he observed that the American public had in some way conceived the idea that the human figure could be standardised. His diet was as follows:

Breakfast
Half an orange, two eggs, one piece of dry toast, coffee
    sweetened with saccharin and two tablespoons of thin
    cream, and one small cube of butter.

Lunch
A slice of lean meat, peas or string beans to the amount of
    two tablespoons, one half-head of lettuce with a little
    French dressing.

Dinner
Clear bouillon, two slices of lean meat, spinach or carrots,
    one half-head lettuce with French dressing, half an
    orange, tea sweetened with saccharin, a quarter of a cup
    of milk, a slice of thin bread toast and a small cube of
    butter.

One should lose, he said, about two pounds a week on this regimen. Anticipating that his readers would be surprised and think his diets contained twice as much as they usually ate, Fishbein was confident that, though varied, his diets had each been chosen with an exact knowledge of what they provided in calories and essential food substances. One must eat well and properly while dieting, 'remember it is not safe to reduce more rapidly'. Dietary experts, he continued, now estimated food values in 100-calorie portions and the way to reduce was to find out how many calories one spent each day and then to eat 500 calories less a day than you spent. When people first began to diet they often felt the pain of hunger and he encouraged them to drink plenty of water and cut down on salts, spices and condiments because they stimulated the flow of gastric juice and increased the appetite. When reducing weight strenuously, the patient should keep in close contact with their doctor so that he could look out for any alarming symptoms and stop the dieting before it did any serious harm.

The main problem was that appetites and desires were capricious. They required study. While savages ate ants and puppy dogs with relish, Eskimos licked their chops over blubber, Mexicans liked hot spices and chilli con carne and Scandinavians ate fish, the average American diet, wrote Fishbein, consisted of pie, ham and eggs and pork and beans. And Americans were getting fat, making them rich pickings for the quack-diet faddists. One of the widely promoted food fads of the time was the Hay diet. This diet did not, 'as many people imagine, emphasize the eating of hay and cereals' but was named after Dr William Hay (1866–1940) whose *Medical Millennium* of 1927 incorporated Fletcher's system of mastication. It reappeared with a bit of a fanfare in the 1980s as the Beverly Hills Diet, illustrating just how these diets feed off each other and spawn revised versions.

Hay himself was overweight and his method advocated careful chewing and a diet based on combining specific foods that, he maintained, could lead to a healthier life and a significantly more slender body. The Hay dieter avoided acidosis (an increased acidity in the blood and body tissues) something that was said to lead directly to fat, by eating starches separately from proteins, and both of these were eaten separately from fruits. Henry Ford, for one, ate this monotrophic diet, taking only fruits at breakfast, starches at lunch and proteins at dinner. To Fishbein, this food combination plan depended on the completely erroneous idea that starches were digested only in the mouth and proteins only in the stomach (making it difficult to digest them at the same time). The idea was ridiculous and without scientific foundation, wrote Fishbein scathingly: it was well understood that starches were mixed with saliva and their digestion, which began in the mouth, was continued in the stomach.

Hay's retreat in the mid-1930s, in the Poconos, Pennsylvania, was called Hay-ven and his book, *Health via Food* (1929), was, according to Fishbein, 'mostly misinformation'. For lunch (starch and sugars), the Hay Diet allowed watercress soup, vegetables in casserole, and then sour cream waffles with maple syrup, and for dinner (proteins and acids) celery soup, mousse of lobster and tomato and lettuce salad. It also relied on salads of vegetables 'prepared according to fancy formulas' and carrying names such as the Fountain of Youth Salad, Pale Moon Cocktail, Easter Bunny Salad, Startled Chicken and Parcel Post Asparagus. And there were 'many directions for torturing carrots into funny shapes'. Fishbein considered these fads for food-combination diets as dangerous and absurd; and as responsible for weakening the confidence of the American people in their diets and their foods generally. The idea that not mixing proteins and carbohydrates was the route to health was disproved by the many generations of Americans who had grown up on meat and potatoes.

Doctors worried that some reduction diets involved only a counting of calories and failed to take into account the body's need for vitamins and mineral salts. Many popular reducing diets, including the Hollywood 18-day diet, the milk menus and other 'similar performances', allowed just 500 to 800 calories a day instead of 1,100 or 1,200, which was the absolute minimum thought compatible with maintaining good health. Women from all over the country flocked to milk farms to try the milk menu, the newest fad. They subsisted for varying periods on milk, orange juice and soup, the milk sometimes being taken in the form of acidophilous milk, lactic acid milk or even the thin yoghurt-like substance known in some parts of the world as 'clabber'. Many regarded such a diet as dangerous because it brought about weight reduction far too rapidly and did not provide sufficient mineral salts, especially iron, to sustain the blood in a normal healthful condition. In the late 1930s, wrote Fishbein, one saw women 'who are haggard and sallow, wandering about in a weakened condition, but still rather proud of the fact that they have taken off in a short period of time anywhere from 10 to 15 pounds. One sees the same women a month later with 10 to 15 pounds restored on those parts of the body on which they would rather have it absent, and nothing to show for their experiment but disappointment and some loss of health.'

Men, he thought, were more active physically for a longer period of time, spent more time in the open air, ate more proteins and fewer sugars, and were less likely to try dieting just to look better, whereas women, as they had babies and got older, had a special tendency to get fat and so to go on diets. It seemed to him that women and girls would often reduce their first meal of the day to just fruit juice and coffee, 'and those who are reducing stringently may even eliminate the fruit juice'. The effect this had on their looks was, he believed, a definite disorder of the human body. Being too skinny could also, of course, be due to over-activity of the thyroid, chain-smoking, nervous exhaustion or lack of sleep, as well as going on the fad crash diets which made women obsessive and likely to resort to enemas, strong cathartics and dangerous over-the-counter obesity cures.

On the subject of Fletcherism, Fishbein lamented that 'whole families could be seen seated at breakfast carefully counting each movement of the jaws to make certain that the number agreed with what Fletcher thought was correct. Obviously there was no scientific basis for any such performance.' Fletcherism itself had passed into the 'limbo of forgotten dietetic fallacies', even though most diet books were still advocating careful chewing of each mouthful of food. Fishbein thought that vegetarianism had developed as a cult at around the same time as Fletcherism (though we have seen the former discussed by eighteenth-century writers), even though meat was now a safe and clean food and had particular values for a healthy body. He thought it interesting that practically every religious belief system had some prohibitive notion relating to foods and their preparation yet the human stomach knew nothing of religion or belief, and sometimes it was 'simply a desire on the part of the person concerned to be different from everybody else, and in that way to acquire a feeling of superiority'. There were courses that dieters could take on auto-intoxication (still very popular today as detox regimens), 'a misnomer if ever there was one' and wholly unscientific, based on the argument that the body became blocked with undigested and decaying food material, an utter untruth in his opinion. As for the Graham System, this was based entirely on a laxative effect. Graham crackers, Graham flour and Graham bread were just loosening roughage, all nothing but 'horse food', coarse and unappetising.

As a people, Fishbein thought that Americans had been cursed with faddists in general and that theirs was a nation peculiarly prone to cultish ideas and movements: educational cults, faith-healing cults, religious cults, among others, and now this plague of dietary faddists. Peculiar schools of dieting were advertised in circulars and sold to people who just didn't know, or perhaps didn't want to know, the truth about what diet could actually do. Fishbein wanted to educate the public: to make them see that starvation was a serious business, that the body would actually consume itself, and if it went on long enough it would die. He despaired that people seemed to believe in all these fads, diet foods and drinks, the bizarre apparatus, special syringes and other devices for losing weight. Society seemed to be obsessed with weight, bodies, behaviour and vanity. Women, and men, were bombarded with judgemental advice, diet and exercise plans, and lone largely sensible voices, such as Fishbein's, were scarcely audible through the shouting and arm-waving of the diet industry. Fishbein was trying to warn and educate us nearly eighty years ago, yet today's fad-diet industry is bigger and more popular than ever.

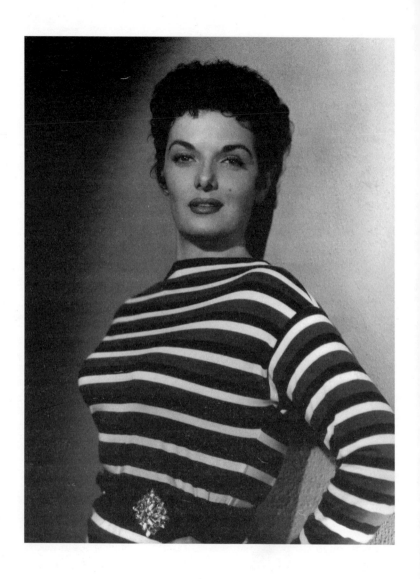

9. Jane Russell's sweater-girl physique was a Hollywood beacon of bodily perfection for the 1940s and 50s. Many diet gurus established themselves within the movie industry recognising it as producing rich pickings among the stars who couldn't 'afford to become fat and unattractive. They know only too well how soon their public will forget them if they do'. And then there was that very public who wanted to emulate their celebrity heroes.

9

Skeletons and Sweater Girls

B Y THE 1940S AND 1950S busts were back in fashion and 'sweater girls' with their trussed-up hour-glass figures were everywhere and all the rage. In America, women wanted to look like Hollywood film stars Lana Turner, Jane Russell and, later, Marilyn Monroe, the first *Playboy* centrefold. In the UK, Diana Dors was big – big, bottle blonde, brassy and busty – though Audrey Hepburn, a role model for the upper classes, slender, discreet and elegant, was also around for contrast. The appetite for dieting and body-shaping was stronger than ever and widely encouraged by the media. Sylvia of Hollywood (1881–1975) (4 ft 8 in. tall and weighing just 100 lb) had been busily massaging the likes of Jean Harlow, Gloria Swanson, Marie Dressler, Norma Shearer, Mae Murray and Ina Claire for years – so that 'fat comes out through the pores like mashed potato through a colander'. But Sylvia, who gave advice in the film fan magazine *Photoplay*, was rumoured to have caused the first Hollywood induced death-by-diet. She recommended a diet of spinach, liver, whole-wheat toast and steamed vegetables, much like the Hollywood 18-day diet. She also told slimmers to make sure that they had a pair of scales in their bathrooms, 'just to put the fear of God in you'.

But Benjamin Gayelord Hauser (1895–1984) was the real Hollywood diet guru of the moment. The medical profession, especially Fishbein, reserved particular contempt for this wealthy, health-food dietician to the stars. Hauser was all over the press, written about almost as much as the starlets he advised, and was referred to as a nationally known, famous Viennese expert on food science. He was actually a charismatic, handsome, 'youngish man with a flashy smile and a broken accent', who 'wears his hair in a permanent wave'. His doctorate was not as permanent as his hair, however, and had to be dropped after an investigation by the American Medical Association. He wasn't even Viennese, let alone any sort of expert, but he had plenty of elaborate diets including the eliminative feeding system, the mending diet, the vitality diet, the transition diet, the cosmetic diet (of sulphur-rich foods), an iron-rich cocktail of spinach, parsley and citrus juice for a beautiful skin, and the zigzag diet which advised a morning purge of Epsom salts and an evening dose of senna. In this last diet most of the weight loss was due to commonly available salts and cathartics which Hauser was selling under his own expensive brand name. His whole system of diets was, according to Fishbein, 'based on misconceptions and fallacies and it [was] dangerous to the public to follow these notions'. Hauser was, he complained, a con-man selling diets to gullible people.

Hauser's books are written in the tone of a self-styled prophet come to bestow upon his adoring female disciples the truth and the way of their proper and only calling: to be beautiful. His book, *Eat and Grow Beautiful* (London, 1939), written at a point in history when you might imagine the world had more on its mind than this, described what he proclaimed to be a new and simple design for living. He claimed that his regimen had been followed religiously by the 'smart women, the leaders in fashion and society' who had discovered the answer to everything in Hauser's Cosmetic diet, and they were proclaiming it to be 'the cornerstone on which they had built new beauty – new vitality – new happiness'. These women, he wrote with undisguised self-congratulation and a beady eye on the market, had made of his 'teachings a vogue which others clamour to follow'. Who would want to be left out? Who would dare?

After all, according to Hauser, beauty, for those women who were lucky enough to possess it, was a thing to be cherished but to 'those less fortunate beings who aspire to it [it was] a goal towards which they continuously strive'. It is the same old line that women have always been sold: they could be better, younger, more loved, if they only bought whatever lotion or potion or system was on offer. Hauser had set himself up in Hollywood because he understood the power of the movie industry and knew that so many diets originated there because 'most of our high-priced movie stars are living in constant fear of losing their attractiveness and thereby their popularity … they simply can't afford to become fat and unattractive. They know only too well how soon their "public" will forget them if they do!' No beauty aid was too expensive, 'no regimen too drastic for these lovely ladies of the screen' – and so, too, of course, for the masses of ordinary women in the street who wanted desperately to be like them.

One of Hauser's lovers, the immaculate Greta Garbo, had him to thank for manufacturing her slim, androgynous elegance. She had slavishly followed his directions, sliding narrowly about on the big screen as a long-running silent advertisement for the benefits of salads and juices. The result was that women every-where took to serious dieting and vigorous exercise regimens to achieve the figure of an adolescent boy. Public demand for films seemed insatiable – by the 1920s the Hollywood movie industry was already worth over $2 billion – and the parallel demand for physically 'perfect' actors was (and still is) an impossibly chal-lenging requirement. Indeed, the movie world so influenced the perceptions of both body shape and character that, in 1924, a Dr James S. McLester had been moved to write in the *Journal of the American Medical Association* that, 'A fat face has a monstrous uniformity. No theatrical producer would hire a plump actress to mirror the real depths of the human soul.'

Hauser's first serious students, as he called them, were movie stars and actresses, then women who had the money and the time to devote to beauty culture, and finally, as he noted, 'it seems that women the world over are willing and anxious to become beautiful' because 'there is real tragedy in fat'. Fat women, he said, were living only half a life, their flesh bloated and their spirits sagged. Being fat was a crime committed against the self and it forced you to live in a world of dreams since the pleasurable realities were so far beyond your reach. Sleep, in these circumstances, became a paradise, the one desire in life – Hauser seemed to suggest that such women would rather be dead than fat, or even rather dead than worried about fat. For fat, and the fear of it, destroyed personal and domestic happiness: who, he asked, could 'estimate how much marital unhappiness was due to the fact that the slim and lovely bride becomes in a few short years a stout, ungainly matron? Who can say how many charming young girls turn into old maids because of the cruel handicap of excess weight? The overweight person may joke about her avoirdupois, even try to laugh it off, but nevertheless every time she looks in the mirror there is a pang of pain. Yet she can become as slim as the slender woman she envies if she at once makes up her mind to it and goes about it in the right way.' Hauser's duplicitous offer of salvation from the very distress he was causing is quite sickening to read.

Still, he pandered to his 'students', telling them that they needed intelligence and perseverance to be successfully slim: there was no short cut, you had to do the job yourself. Massage could be effective – you could have yourself slapped and rolled for weeks and lose several pounds, but those pounds would come back unless the food you ate was specially selected not to create fat. One didn't need to depend on drugs, such as dinitrophenol, which worked only by burning off weight and endangering health and life itself. There was just one simple and effective way to lose weight, according to Hauser, and that was to follow his diets.

This didn't mean starving yourself, which was neither as simple as people might think, nor, more importantly, remotely sane. Fasting was a health hazard in Hauser's opinion, as it flooded the body with waste poisons and very often led to headaches and acidosis. Hauser claimed that his plan was not only 'scientific' but was free from hard work. It worked to re-educate people's tastes away from starchy and sugary foods and 'to build up a desire for the cleansing, vitalizing foods which spell slenderness and health'. Simple fundamentals and rules never fail, he wrote, if applied conscientiously. And, presumably, paid for.

Time and time again, Hauser said, he had seen a tendency to overeat all the wrong foods. His 'lovely ladies of the screen' were given slenderising fruit juices before they dashed off to the studio for the day's work and ordinary women should follow this celebrity example. (Now, of course, celebrities flog us their diet and exercise regimens directly, although gurus still have their place. James Duigan, for example, styles himself as the founder of Bodyism, 'a unique nutritional and personal training system'. Duigan has models and film stars among his clientele, of course, including Elle Macpherson and Hugh Grant, but there's no reason why you can't buy into it too. Duigan claims he can get you into shape fast and without much effort. Does this sound familiar? The first step is to follow his simple 14-day Clean and Lean Kick-start plan. 'You must believe you can do this,' he says. 'It doesn't matter how often you have failed in the past.')

But back to the 1930s. For breakfast, one should have only

fruit or fruit juices; for lunch, just a salad, for bulk and roughage, precious minerals and vitamins. Obviously, Hauser realised that these intelligent women would probably all be crying, 'What about our husbands? Surely a man cannot have just a salad for lunch', to which he replied, why not? Some of his followers were, he claimed, the ablest leaders of industry. Men, as we know, would be eating the salad for efficiency's sake, certainly not to be considered beautiful. It was simply very 'good for work!!!' Anyway, having been careful so far you could now have almost anything you wanted for dinner, as long as you remembered this: 'FIRST, EAT WHAT YOU NEED, THEN EAT WHAT YOU WANT'. Beginning with a vegetable juice cocktail or salad, you might go on with meat and one or two cooked vegetables. In place of bread or potatoes you should eat his 'appetite spoilers' which were radishes, onions, celery sticks, carrot sticks, or small bunches of raw cauliflower, all chilled first. Then perhaps a large bowl of fresh fruit, fruit compote or water ice for dessert, which would not only melt away those superfluous pounds but would 'actually take years away from your appearance!' Meat in excess was a weight hazard, so lean cuts only – never fried, always broiled. Fish was the less fattening option. He approved of exercise (but doubted how many women actually did it); walking or dancing were best. Drinking too much water was a definite 'weight builder', so one should stay away from spices that could make you thirsty. Instead, stick to water with lemon juice – between shots on the set Hauser's starlets could be seen sipping this cooling, tart drink. Above all there should be nothing unreasonable, nothing tyrannical about a reducing diet and, if you happened to feel tired while on one, you might find his 'pickme-up' cocktails especially helpful.

In a particularly chilling anecdote Hauser happily demonstrated the insidious nature of his business: 'A friend of mine,' he wrote, 'a successful director in Hollywood, has a little girl of who

I am very fond. One day I visited this friend and being left alone for a few moments with the child I asked her, "And what will you do, dear, when you are as big as your mother?" This very modern child replied unhesitatingly and with an absolutely serious face: "Diet!" That so many of us, he wrote, 'have misshapen, almost grotesque bodies is due, in the great majority of cases, to our own indifference or ignorance'. Fortunately, it was never too late for the irredeemably fat and ugly. With scientific knowledge, proper tools and good materials Hauser would help you 'smooth out those bulging places and attain streamlined effects instead of exaggerated and dangerous curves'. No matter how old or misshapen you were he could help you regain the figure you had when you were Sweet Sixteen, still there though 'hidden under the soft, ugly rolls of flabby flesh'.

Although science wasn't really Hauser's strong point he did believe that endocrinology, good old scientific 'Gland Magic', could help. And it had to be magic because how else could the over-secretion of a gland turn the classic profile of a Barrymore into something which might well have come out of the latest wild-animal thriller? Gland Magic could overcome the 'Handicaps to Beauty'. Dysfunctional glands ruined beauty and health and caused constipation, giving a woman sallow skin, dull eyes and brittle, dry and lifeless hair. The delayed food putrified, the body absorbed the poisons and the only thing more dangerous than this was the means by which many people took to get rid of it. Becoming panicky, they took pill after pill, laxative after laxative, and kept on until they had developed the 'laxative-a-day' habit that enslaved them for life. The real and only cure was, again, one of Hauser's diets, plus a little bit of Fletcherism (even if it had ludicrous aspects).

Hauser was no fool. His success lay in his charisma and in his use of basic common sense – as well as smart PR. He warned against food faddism even as he promoted it: but he was different, his way was the truth! 'A hundred different cults clamor for our attention,' he wrote. 'Hysterical, fanatical shouting! Sweeping, all-inclusive generalizations! Grotesque theories one day, their repudiation the next! No wonder so many of us throw up our hands in despair! There is one rule that holds – and that is … Stay away from extremes. I wish I could write this in letters ten feet high!' If you remove the manipulative and anxiety-inducing smoke and mirrors, you find that Hauser's diets were based on common sense. But he couldn't sell that to people who already had it, could he? In a later book, *Look Younger, Live Longer* (he knew his market), published in 1951, Hauser argued that there was no such thing as a 'stylish stout'. Flatten it, he cajoled, strengthen it, 'make it your aim in life to keep your muscles so strong and elastic that you can free yourself permanently from that one-piece harness called the corset. Your own muscular corset is the best of all undergarments.' Despite Hauser's advice, women in the 1950s and 1960s were again squeezing themselves into tortuous but fashionable body-shaping undergarments. The Vanishette, a 'Figure Slimming Miracle of Paris!', featured a Magic Lastex Waist Band that would 'INSTANTLY Vanish 4 INCHES OFF YOUR WAIST!' In 1956 American *Vogue* ran a piece on women and waistlines, and the proof that they wanted them was the $6,000,000 they spent every year on the famous waist-making 'Merry Widow', a brassiere-and-waist-cincher combination. In Paris, *Vogue* carried an advertisement for a corset for every age and figure problem, to 'dissimulate cellulite and to appear thin when one is not'.

The resurgence of this market had a lot to do with the resumption of the rubber business after the Second World War. When the Malayan rubber plantations were captured by the Japanese in 1941, all synthetic rubber was used for gas masks and not inessential goods such as corsets; the corset factories were pulled into the war effort and began to manufacture parachute harnesses and chinstraps for helmets. When peace broke out they went back to reviving and capitalising on the underwear market. *Life* magazine began discussing 'waist pinchers', new, tiny corsets that squeezed waists and emphasised 'full hips and a high bosom', and arguing that this development was bad news for the American male who would find himself paying for foundations that 'will present a Maginot Line of elastic and steel' every time he 'sneaks an arm around an attractive waist'.

Louise Paine Benjamin, an associate editor of the *Ladies' Home Journal* who wrote on beauty, health and exercise, published a piece in her magazine in 1940 that encouraged girls to 'take an interest in their appearance when they are very young' and to 'resist the three S's: Sundaes, Sodas, and Second Helpings'. Benjamin had her three daughters, then all under fifteen years old, doing posture exercises to prevent them acquiring 'protruding derrieres and tummy bulges'. She also wrote a book that appeared in 1941, entitled *Why Men Like Us: Your Passport to Charm*. By the 1950s, quite blatant advertisements for RyKrisp appeared, helpfully informing anyone who hadn't quite got the picture that 'Nobody Loves a Fat Girl'. The girls' magazine, *Seventeen*, was telling its young readers that fat was a medical problem, that they should think carefully about what they were eating and try keeping to a diet of between 1,200 and 1,800 calories a day. Delving into the psychology of eating it instructed them not to 'pamper your blues' with comfort food.

There was a growing emphasis and interest in the psychology of eating and in 'the importance of the patient's whole personality', as opposed to just what she ate. Dr Margaret Mead, who was the Executive Secretary on the Committee on Food and Habits for the National Research Council in Washington DC, pointed out that this made all sorts of new demands on doctors and dieticians as they looked more closely at specific food behaviour and special diets for the sick, which were themselves 'concomitants of deep-seated personality distortions and over-emphases'. In post-war America, overweight women were generally denounced as lazy and undisciplined, but now this generally accepted truism was backed up by the nation's psychiatrists who pronounced that they had exposed the fat person for what she really was – miserable, self-indulgent and lacking in self-control. This quite ridiculous and contemptible woman was likely to compound her folly by accusing her husband of being 'supercritical' which 'makes her too nervous to plan menus or to shop properly (she would be a lot more nervous if she knew her husband is running around with his slim secretary because his wife is so fat and unattractive)'.

It wasn't all one way, though, and men and boys were also coming under increasing pressure about their body shape and size. Elmer Wheeler's *Fat Boy's Book: How Elmer Lost 40 Pounds in 80 Days* was serialised in the General Features newspaper syndicate in 1950, and it reached an estimated thirty million American readers. Wheeler had dieted down from an enormous 230 pounds on 1,500 calories a day – though his 'day' lasted 72 hours. The book sold 112,000 copies in the year following its publication, and he received more than three million letters in response to his diet plan. About 90,000 hopeful dieters bought his dieting slide rule, a calorie intake measure, from the *Chicago Daily News*. This helpfully pointed out that human skeletons and unhappy lovers were able to live on 300 calories a day, barflies and somnambulists could exist on 1,700, models and bums on 2,100, mothers of triplets and three-day poker players on 3,200, gluttons on 4,500 and, finally, grave diggers needed up to 5,000 calories. In 1952 Wheeler published again, this time a confessional follow-up called the *Fat Boy's Downfall and How Elmer Learned to Keep It Off* in which he wrote that the minimum number of calories needed was 900 a day, that living on 1,200 was No Fun, 1,500 was Safe Reducing, then at 1,800 came the

Kitchen Sneaks, those on 2,100 were Cheaters, those on 2,400 were Backsliders, you were a rank Self-deceiver at 2,700, a Fat Boy on 3,000, a Glutton on 3,300, and those who consumed 3,600 calories were the ultimate Hopeless Cases. The Fat Boy phenomenon was extremely popular and spin-offs included a new tune called 'The Fat Boy Bounce' put out by the Mills Music Company, and 'The Fat Boy Cigar' sold by Bering Cigars.

Physical culture for men had also become big business. Successful bodybuilders on both sides of the Atlantic such as Eugen Sandow (1867–1925), Jørgen Peter Müller (1866–1938) and Thomas Inch (1881–1963) had been promoting exercise regimens for a taut, manly muscularity for decades, but it was Charles Atlas (1893–1972) who really began the craze among Joe Public. Atlas, born Angelo Siciliano in Calabria, Italy, had emigrated to Brooklyn, New York with his seamstress mother when he was a child of ten and it was on a Coney Island beach that the legend began. As a teenager weighing in at a mere ninety-seven pounds, Angelo was trying to impress a pretty girl when he was literally put down by a much sturdier young man. The girl went off with the other guy. It is a story with which many young men would identify. Angelo transformed himself into a living god, after a statue he had seen at the Brooklyn Museum, with a self-devised exercise and diet regimen. He transformed his fortunes, too, and became, according to *Physical Culture Magazine*, the World's Most Perfectly Developed Man, who could pull railroad cars along their tracks, tow boats through New York Harbor and who was soon handling an enormously profitable mail-order company by promising to turn feeble weaklings into muscle-bound men. It has been estimated that up to six million young men bought into his regimen over some sixty years.

His theory of physical development came to him, he said, when he was watching the lions at the Prospect Park Zoo: they didn't lift weights, they just stretched their bodies to achieve their muscular beauty and strength. Angelo set about pushing one set of his muscles against another and apparently doubled his weight in just one year so that, by the time he was nineteen years old, he was a professional Coney Island strong man, standing 5 ft 10 in. tall, weighing 180 lb, with a 47 in. chest, a 32 in. waist, a 17 in. neck, 14 in. forearms and 24 in. thighs. He renamed himself Charles Atlas and modelled for heroic works of art, including the statue of George Washington of the Washington Square Arch, Dawn of Glory in Prospect Park, and Alexander Hamilton at the US Treasury in Washington. *Physical Culture Magazine* cancelled their bodybuilding competition at Madison Square Garden when they realised that no one else but Atlas was ever going to win it. He was an obvious choice for the part of Tarzan in the Hollywood films, but he decided he didn't want to leave Brooklyn.

The Charles Atlas business really took off when he joined forces with an advertising man who coined the term 'Dynamic Tension' for his exercises. It was advertised in every magazine by the late 1930s, and 60,000 men a year were shelling out $30 a time for their Charles Atlas Way of Life. And it really was everywhere: it is said that when an order arrived from India, purportedly from Mahatma Gandhi, Atlas sent back a specially devised lesson plan and would not take any money for it, saying 'Poor little chap, he's nothing but a bag of bones.' Another story tells of an anthropologist in Africa coming across a Bantu village that had set up a shrine to Atlas, adorned with advertisements torn out of *Argosy*, the first American pulp magazine that was aimed at the boys' adventure market.

Young men were not only being encouraged to shape their bodies; Atlas had an eye on their minds too. They were encouraged to 'avoid all dissipations and injurious habits you know to be wrong', to think high and beautiful thoughts, not to go to burlesque shows, and to understand that a sound body and sound mind go together. His critics included the Federal Trade Commission, who continually suggested he was nothing but a fraud. Others who tried to ruin his reputation with scandal found none. The whole world looked up to him, said Atlas, who took it all extremely seriously: it was a great responsibility being the 'most ideal specimen of the human body'. 'You only have one body,' he wrote, 'you can't go to the store and get another one.' In his seventies, Atlas was still exercising rigorously, walking, swimming and stretching, and he continued to complain about the way people ate. They were all eating 'dead food', he railed. 'Everything is artificial! Not enough Vitamin A!' Atlas, the self-tortured ideal of American manhood, blamed American women, accusing them of being plain selfish: 'Mothers going here and there, wearing pants like a man, showing their backsides to people,' he ranted 'What is this? They should be home cooking real food and feeding their families instead of out showing their backsides ... kids today look bad because their mothers feed them pop and crackers.' That easiest and most conspicuous of targets, the uppity, slothful, fat American female, took the blame again for the dissipation of the nation.

Some researchers did manage to come up with diet plans that were satisfied with giving information and avoided attacking any particular group. Dorothea Turner of the American Dietetic Association published her *Handbook of Diet Therapy* in 1946, under the University of Chicago Press, to 'maintain, or to bring the patient to, a state of nutritive efficiency'. Even in the 1940s, researchers were still utilising insurance company tables: Turner's figures were lifted from the 1943 Metropolitan Life Insurance Company's Statistical Bureau and their Table of Ideal Weights for men, women, children and adolescents. A woman of 5 ft 4 in. (in her shoes) with a small frame, for example, should weigh between 116 and 125 lb dressed in her everyday clothes. If she was of medium frame she should be between 124 and 132 lb, and of large frame between 131 and 142 lb. To achieve these ideals Turner produced a low-calorie diet, a modification of usual diet patterns, so that the number of calories the dieter was allowed in the course of a day was consistently below the number needed. In this way, the diet would lead to a loss of body fat while the necessary proteins, minerals and vitamins would remain at the required nutritional levels. Her 'moderate reduction programme' ranged from between 1,000 and 1,500 calories for women and between 1,500 and 2,000 for men, and if this resulted in 'a daily deficit of approximately 1,200 calories per day, or 8,400 calories per week, a loss of 930 g or 2 lb of fat (1 g of fat yields approximately 9 calories) per week may be expected'. The diet was as follows:

Breakfast
Half a grapefruit or 1 orange.
1 egg.
1 slice toast or bread.
Coffee or tea if desired, with milk from allowance.
4 level teaspoons of butter or margarine for entire day in cooking and on the bread.
Note: two level teaspoons of sugar or jelly or honey may be substituted for 1 teaspoon of butter or margarine.

Noon Meal
2 oz of meat (boil, broil or roast).
2 vegetables, as in fat-free vegetable soup, vegetable-juice cocktail, salad, or cooked vegetables.
Fruit (e.g. 1 medium apple).
1 glass milk.
1 slice bread.
Tea or coffee, if desired.

Evening Meal
Same as noon, with the addition of one small potato.

If you had to go out to eat in a restaurant, Turner sensibly instructed you to select only plain-cooked, low-calorie foods, salad and fruit, advising that excess calories that went to fat could be worked off with exercise. This may have been easier said than done, however. In *How to Control Your Weight* (1942), Hazel M. Hauck had calculated that, with 3,600 calories to the pound of flesh, a dieter climbing the 2,240 steps of the Empire State Building would probably lose only half a pound. To work off a whole pound the dieter would have to lay 14,731 bricks or scrape dirty laundry across a washboard 2,100 times an hour for 28 hours straight. A 150-pound person dancing the mazurka full-on for an hour might lose no more than a pound; a pat of butter is the equivalent of climbing the steps inside the Washington Monument; and to lose the effects of just one doughnut would necessitate you conducting an orchestra for two and a half hours. Even one measly Graham Cracker needed more than a half-mile walk to work it off your hips.

Sylvester Graham (1794–1851) himself, inventor of the famous cracker, maintained that the stomach is a liar pretending to be concerned with the digestive system, whereas in reality it is in the pay of the nervous system. The same message is being repeated today, too. Since 1985, the average man in Britain has burned off 1,380 calories a day through exercise, and the average woman 950 calories and the commonly accepted idea that we live more sedentary lives these days is flawed. Physical activity has remained the same for at least the past twenty-five years yet we have got fatter and fatter because we eat more and more high-calorie foods. An obese person with a body mass index of 35 could reach a more healthy weight, and a BMI of 22, it is claimed, by reducing their calorie intake by one third, the equivalent to around five hours of exercise a day. Eating less of certain foods is apparently the more realistic answer to losing weight.

There was still, during this period, plenty of room in the market for gurus peddling less than scientific diet plans. The first overtly Christian slimming book, Charlie W. Shedd's *Pray Your Weight Away*, was published in 1957. Shedd (1915–2004) was pastor of the Memorial Drive Presbyterian Church of Houston and, having shed his own 100 pounds of fat, was preaching to his plump parishioners that, 'we fatties are the only people on earth who can weigh our sin'. God, according to Shedd, had dreamed man to be thin, so fat was a matter of sin and redemption. Deborah Pierce, who wrote *I Prayed Myself Slim* (1960), had experienced some sort of epiphany over gluttony. 'Suddenly,' she wrote, 'I had a strange and exultant feeling as I remembered something. It was as if I were on the verge of a miracle.' If gluttony was a sin then perhaps God would help her overcome it. So she prayed: 'Almighty God, when things seem too much for me, and my stomach begins to rebel, it is only through Thy presence and guidance that I may overcome my weakness.' She attended Prayer-Diet Clubs – 'The Lord is my Shepherd. He will lead me away from food and gluttony into the higher paths of life' – and by 1960 was a successful fashion model. The Reverend H. Victor Kane, thinking along the same lines, published *Devotions for Dieters* in 1967, and included a little prayer:

I promise not to sit and stuff
But stop when I have had enough.
Amen.

In 1972, having sat on the board of a psychiatric hospital, Pastor Charlie Shedd followed up his earlier entreaties with another book, *The Fat is in Your Head*, in which he proclaimed 'Scratch a fat man and you will find a neurotic.' In the mid-1970s, the journalist Ellen Goodman remarked that, 'eating had become the last bona fide sin left in America' as she filed reports on revivalist diet workshops led by the Overeaters Victorious movement who referred to the text of John 3:30, 'He must increase, but I must decrease' or, as Joan Cavanaugh wrote in 1976, *More of Jesus, Less of Me*. Marie Chapian, in her book *Free to be Thin* (1979), co-authored with Neva Coyle (the founder and director of Overeaters Victorious and president of Neva Coyle Ministries), wrote that 'Jesus died on the cross for me to set me free from the addiction to wrong foods.' Carol Showalter, meanwhile, came up with the 3D diet based on Diet, Discipline and Discipleship. Showalter was married to a senior minister of the Presbyterian church in Rochester, New York, and founded 3D after a ten-year struggle with her 167 pounds, taking her cue from Luke 9:23 – 'If any man would come after me, let him deny himself and take up his cross daily and follow me.' Evelyn Kliewer, in *Freedom from Fat* (1977), drew on Ephesians 6:12: 'For we wrestle not against flesh and blood, but against principalities, against powers, against the rulers of the darkness of this world, against spiritual wickedness in high places.'

The Jesus System of Weight Control promised freedom and empowerment because 'With Jesus, you can't lose – or should I say, All you can do is lose!' and 'Jesus went to the cross so that His people no longer need be the victims of compulsive acts.' In 1978 Dr C. S. Lovett came out with *Help Lord: The Devil Wants Me Fat!* asking, 'If you were the devil, wouldn't you seek to penetrate lives at a point where you'd never be suspected? Sure. Well, what is more innocent than food? With Christians THANKING GOD for what they eat, what neater way to slip into their lives than with EXTRA spoonfuls of delicious food … Subtle, right?' Lovett obviously couldn't match the devil for subtlety. His ideological stance was an important diet tool that he shared with many other Christian diet writers – and it was a mixed blessing if you failed to lose weight or keep it off.

Private spas, too, whose own approach often verged on the religious, continued to spring up, including enterprises like the Pritikin Longevity and Spa Center in Miami whose founder, Nathan Pritikin (1915–85), developed a health programme after being diagnosed with heart disease in 1958, at the age of forty-one. Pritikin, who had no medical training, undertook research on which populations lived longest, such as the Japanese and Chinese, and came up with a diet plan packed with vegetables, fruit and lean protein, and daily exercise. After two years he had lost a significant amount of weight and greatly improved his health, and in the 1970s he opened his residential centre to the paying, plump public. His regimen is familiar and simple: regular exercise and a diet of whole foods such as fruit, vegetables, whole grains, seafood and some lean meat. Now even the American government includes Pritikin advisers on its dietary public health advice board.

In the 1960s, products and ideas that had previously only seen the light of day in medical publications began to appear on national television and in the press. One such product was the diet formula Metrecal, made by Mead Johnson and Co., which was advertised vaguely as 'not exactly a drug product, not exactly a food product'. It soon had competition from other large companies and their products, including Sears Roebuck's Bal-Cal, Quota by Quaker Oats, Korvette's Kor-Val, Jewel Tea Company's Diet-Cal, Ovaltine's Minvitine and Pet Milk's Sego. Combined sales of Sego and Metrecal came to more than $450 million in 1965. In the following decade the press was swamped with adverts for Doctor's Diet Reducing Tabs, the Sauna Slim Suit, Vib-a-Way Tummy Toner, the Body Taper-Trim Shirt and the Trim-a-Bod Slimmer (by the end of the decade in America there were fifty-eight products registered under the name 'Trim'

– Trim Beer, Trim-Thi, Trimcycle, Trimfit hosiery …), and the 3-Way Diet Program that rather worryingly claimed to 'LITER-ALLY MELT THE FAT OFF YOUR BODY LIKE A BLOW-TORCH WOULD MELT BUTTER'.

Many of these slimming foods and drinks contained artificial sweeteners. Saccharin, a substance entirely without calories yet some three to five hundred times as sweet as common sugar, was accidentally discovered in 1879 by Constantin Fahlberg at Johns Hopkins University in Baltimore. It was first used as food preservative before becoming popular during the First World War when sugar shortages hit, and soon saccharin was being sold for table and cooking use for dieters and diabetics. President Theodore Roosevelt had been advised by his doctors to use it and, when his Pure-Food-and-Drug investigator, Dr Harvey W. Wiley, told him that it might well be dangerous to health he retorted, 'Anybody who says saccharin is injurious to health is an idiot.' In 1910 a national committee of scientists agreed that small amounts were 'acceptable' and it was not until 1951 that the first reports appeared suggesting saccharin was a carcinogen. By 1970 cyclamates had been banned as carcinogens, and the following year the FDA removed saccharin from the list of food additives generally recognised as safe. Still, by 1981 the American domestic market for sweeteners was worth about $2 billion and about a third of all Americans were regularly consuming them in diet products or using sweeteners such as Sucaryl and Sweet 'N Low – in the mid-eighties Sweet 'N Low was being used by more than 29 million people more than 30 million times a day. Another type of sweetener, aspartame – brand name NutraSweet – was discovered in 1965 by a lab working on an ulcer treatment and was approved by the FDA in 1981. This nutritive sweetener (that is a sweetener with some calorific value) was promoted in television commercials as a 'sweetening ingredient that isn't fat-tening. A sweetening ingredient that isn't artificial like saccharin.

Isn't bad for your teeth. Tastes just like sugar. And sounds just too good to be true.' Twenty years later anecdotal reports that also thought it was too good to be true led to the British Food Standards Agency calling for a review of earlier safety assessments. The market for proprietary slimming foods and drinks is constantly under strict review because of their artificial ingredients, and diet drugs have to be just as avidly policed.

In the 1960s, a variety of 'mother's little helpers' filled medicine cabinets in homes everywhere. Most were amphetamine-based and available in capsule form under anodyne-sounding names but, although these were prone to pilfering, the recreational use of amphetamines was not widespread until cocaine was declared illegal by the US Federal Government in 1914 – though the notion of what is 'recreational' and what 'medical' is perhaps debatable where the use and abuse of slimming drugs are concerned.

Much about these drugs is, in fact, debatable. Take dinitrophenol, a slimming wonder drug once full of magic promise for the too plump. A derivative of benzene and a carcinogenic dyeing agent, dinitrophenol was also used in First World War explosives. It had been noted as an industrial toxin since 1889, slowly poisoning the people who worked with it in the munitions factories. Absorbed through the skin or inhaled as dust or fume, it was not neutralised by the body nor was it easily washed away with liquids. At a high dose a victim could suffer fatal hyperpyremia, which means burning up with an extraordinarily high fever; in low doses it was still very dangerous to diabetics. Dinitrophenol made people feel warm and sweaty and was often accompanied by a bad rash, while some users lost their sense of taste or even went blind. To make matters worse, dieters tended to exceed the recommended dose, perhaps thinking that twice as much means twice as thin and, possibly, twice as fast. Sir Arthur McNalty, who succeeded George Newman as Chief Medical Officer at the

Ministry of Health, considered slimming to be merely a cosmetic concern and suggested that dieters should avoid all slimming drugs and preparations, except on express medical advice. Dinitrophenol especially, he said, should not be taken under any circumstances. The drug was eventually suppressed in 1938 by which point up to 100,000 people in America were swallowing this miracle pill as a quick and easy route to a willowy frame. At a low dose it would increase the metabolism by 50 per cent, and you might lose between two and three pounds a week – not a spectacularly perceptible or divine intervention given the risks involved.

Morris Fishbein had much to say on dinitrophenol in his essay on 'Drug Treatment and Fads'. 'So persistent is the craze for slenderization,' he wrote, 'that women throughout our country indulge in all sorts of dangerous methods of weight reduction. Every six months there is some new fad or some new technique to which women flock in considerable numbers until science shows their fallacy and the harm that these methods cause. In the thirties women everywhere were trying dinitrophenol until eventually cases began to appear in which the use of this drug had brought about cataracts of the eye. There are now a considerable number of women who have paid for their vanity by the loss of sight.' Many slimmers before this had been using thyroid preparations and risking hyperthyroidism which involved a rapid heart beat, irritability of the nervous system and other serious systematic upsets. Still others had used 'patent medicines containing drugs without efficiency and had spent their money without any result, except damage to health'. Now these dangers had just become even more desperate.

A few slimmers lost their lives as well as their flab after taking other drugs, including Formula 37, Slim and Corpu-lean. Slimming pills became even bigger business when dieters who had been using cocaine switched to amphetamines, freely available from the 1930s. Benzedrine was a favourite, an amphetamine originally developed to control narcolepsy and exhaustion, but it was also prescribed for anhedonia, an inability to experience pleasure and a condition of depressive lethargy which could also cause sufferers to overeat in compensation for their emotional restlessness – they could never be satisfied and grew fat. By 1952, more than 60,000 pounds of amphetamines were being produced annually in the United States, enough for nearly 3 billion 10 mg doses. By the summer of 1970, at the peak of the Vietnam War, 8 per cent of all prescriptions were for amphetamines, a figure that doesn't include all the illegal traffic. At least two billion of these prescriptions were for weight loss. The American Medical Association had disapproved of amphetamines for this purpose as early as 1943, but five years later doctors were handing out Dexedrine as the favourite slimming drug, often together with barbiturates to calm the pill-poppers down. But the effects of amphetamines wore off after six to ten weeks so pharmaceutical companies began looking for longer-acting drugs and came up with Tenuate, Preludin, Lucofen and Didrex, 'for the obese patient chained by the habit of overeating', and Biphetamin and Ionamin were given to lessen the link between appetite anxiety and fat. Over-the-counter drugs such as Appedrine, Prolamine, Control and Dexatrim sold in astonishing quantities, and millions of dollars' worth shot off the shelves. One of the ingredients, phenylpropanolamine, a drug also used for cold and hayfever symptoms, was approved by the FDA in 1979 as a safe and mild appetite suppressant but is no longer recommended for use due to risk of haemorrhagic stroke (bleeding into the brain or the tissue surrounding the brain).

The man who devised the famous Mediterranean diet, still advocated today as a means to a long and healthy life, based his work on plain food, good sense and even better evidence. Ancel Keys (1904–2004) was an American physiologist who published

many successful diet and cookery books, written with his wife
Margaret Keys, such as *Eat Well and Stay Well* (1959), *The Benevo-
lent Bean* (1967) and *Eat Well and Stay Well the Mediterranean
Way* (1975). The books were an immediate hit and Keys was soon
appearing on the cover of *Time* magazine as he became known
to the public as 'Mr Cholesterol'. When America entered the
Second World War, Keys was occupied developing army ration
packs and then in studying the effects of starvation on the millions of European war survivors. One of his major discoveries
was to establish a connection between diet and heart disease.
The incidence of heart disease had fallen dramatically in post-
war hungry people, and when an Italian colleague at the World
Health Organization (Keys chaired its first commission on Food
and Agriculture in Rome) remarked to him that this illness
was not a problem in his country, Keys began his Seven Countries Study in which he monitored more than 12,000 men aged
between 40 and 59 from Italy, the Greek islands, Yugoslavia, the
Netherlands, Finland, Japan and the United States. These men
had contrasting dietary patterns but relatively similar work in
rural labouring. It became obvious that for those groups who
ate fat as a large part of every meal – America and Finland –
bloodstream cholesterol was highest and the heart-attack death
rate the greatest. For the men who ate mainly fresh fruit and
vegetables, bread, pasta and lots of olive oil – around the Mediterranean – blood cholesterol was significantly lower and heart
attacks were much more rare. Finns suffered 992 attacks in every
10,000, while Cretans suffered only 9 in every 10,000, and this
motivated the Finnish government to take steps to regulate diets
that cut the cardiovascular mortality by more than half in the
affected communities by the 1990s. Keys himself lived to be
almost 101 years old, dying in 2004 just two months before his
birthday. He was a lifelong adherent of low-fat foods combined
with regular, 'safe, useful exercise' and he remained a powerful

critic of fad diets. In an interview given in 1959 he blamed his country's problem with heart disease on 'the North American habit for making the stomach a garbage disposal unit for a long list of harmful foods'.

Like many others who became diet planners, Keys had lived an eclectic life. When he was still a teenager he had run away from home to collect bat guano in Arizona caves, and he'd also worked in the Colorado goldmines and as a lumberjack. He got married at just nineteen, and divorced quite soon afterwards, and then abandoned a chemistry degree at Berkeley to work aboard a ship travelling to China. He returned to Berkeley and took a degree in economics and political science and then went to work in Woolworth's before taking an MSc in zoology in 1927 and, three years later, a doctorate in oceanography and biology. He also studied in Copenhagen and at King's College, Cambridge where he turned down a post for one at Harvard that allowed him to concentrate on human physiology. He wanted, he wrote, 'to find out what would be the effect of starvation, how long it would last and what would be required to bring them back to normal'. This work was to be published as *The Biology of Human Starvation* (1950), a work still regarded as the best account of the physiological and cognitive effects of starvation in humans.

The Biology of Human Starvation looked into the relationship between diet, metabolism and health. The two-volume work was the result of an experiment on thirty-six conscientious objectors during the Second World War in which Keys explored the relationships between height and weight and diet and blood fats on the incidence of heart attacks. The study involved his group of young, fit and healthy men eating normally for a period before undergoing three months of semi-starvation during which they walked the equivalent of twenty-two miles a week. They then went through a rehabilitation phase. Once on their starvation diet, the young men, who had no history of weight problems and no previous particular interest in food, found that food was all they wanted to talk and read about, and all they dreamed of at night. They became fascinated by cookery and menus and, half way through their three months of semi-starvation, thirteen of them were talking about taking up cookery as a career when the experiment was finally over. Many of the participants, though, found it impossible to stick to the diet, and secretly and impulsively began sneaking in food, then feeling guilty for doing so. They started displaying anxiety and became prone to depression, had difficulty concentrating, and became withdrawn. Two of the men had emotional breakdowns, and another cut off the end of his finger in order to get himself rejected from the experiment. All of them began to see their bodies in a very different light. When the dieting programme ended, their personalities apparently reverted to normal, but some of the group continued to have problems with eating and to be unhappily preoccupied with food. Keys's study revealed just how intense the psychological as well as physiological effects are of drastically reducing the amount you eat, and his work had an influential and lasting effect on the public's attitudes to what they ate and how much exercise they took.

British children of the 1950s were encouraged in the postwar habit of finishing up every scrap of food on their plates. Even now, many of this generation find it hard to leave or throw away food, regardless of whether or not they are full, and are mildly surprised when others do. During the Second World War a 'deprivation' diet of low-fat, low-carbohydrate, high-fibre, small portions was imposed on people in the UK, and the population benefited from a level of health and fitness unsurpassed since then. In America the war led to a shift in the usual eating patterns to a more cosmopolitan diet as population movements exposed people to a wider variety of American foods. Post-war expansion of international trade and returning soldiers, who had been introduced to a variety of foreign foods and cooking methods, also brought change to eating patterns and habits. Food rationing (which ended in America in 1946 but in the UK lasted until midnight on 4 July 1954) and shortages continued to affect the way people ate.

Cultural change was shaping public attitudes to dieting. The 1950s and 1960s were designated the 'Atomic Age', a phrase dreamed up by a *New York Times* journalist who covered the development of the first nuclear weapons and had witnessed the bombing of Nagasaki. The Cold War was established, the Soviets had launched Sputnik 1 in 1957, and public awareness of scientific advances was high. What's this got to do with dieting? We need to think again about the individual body and the body politic, to see how individuals and societies view themselves through the same prism. *Eat Fat and Grow Slim* was published by Richard MacKarness in 1958 and explained how, in the previous ten years, atomic research had helped physiologists unravel biochemical reactions in the human body. Reporting on the use of radioactive isotopes to tag chemical substances in the body, MacKarness (1916–96) told his readers how they could follow their progress and discover information about the metabolism of fats and carbohydrates, substances 'previously shrouded in mystery'. This process gave new insight into a seemingly contradictory fact about excess fat, that is, how some people overate and got fat while others on the same diet did not. This was an observation of long-standing: Boswell, as we saw in Chapter Four, was remarking upon the unfairness of it over two hundred years ago and Lambie addressed it in the 1930s. The two groups, those who put on weight easily and those who did not, were the subject of a study at the Royal Society of Medicine in London in 1950, by Professor Sir Charles Dodds. His experiment took people whose weights had remained constant for years and got them to eat two or three times their usual amount of food. They didn't put on weight but increased their metabolic rate to burn up the extra calories. The group whose weight had fluctuated over time also ate these greater amounts but were found to get fat and had no increase in their metabolism. So, individuals of the same size, doing the same level of activity and eating the same meals responded quite differently to overeating.

MacKarness argued that this well-known phenomenon was routinely ignored by the 'experts' who were producing all the diet books and articles for slimmers. These books were primarily, he thought, about tricking people into eating less while seeming to allow them to eat more. He gave the example of the medical correspondent for the *Times* from 1957: 'It is no use saying,' wrote the journalist, 'as so many women do "But I eat practically nothing". The only answer to this is: No matter how little you imagine you eat, if you wish to lose weight you must eat less. Your reserves of fat are then called on to provide the necessary energy – and you lose weight.' MacKarness regarded this attitude as quite mistaken, heartless, unfortunately very common, and completely out of date. It harked back to the ideas of William Wadd who in 1829 had unscientifically attributed excess fat to indulgence at the table and had recommended eating foods with little nutritive value. And even as recently as 1930 a piece in the *Journal of Clinical Investigation* had firmly stated that, 'Obesity is never directly caused by abnormal metabolism but is always due to food habits not adjusted to the metabolic requirements'; in other words being fat is not caused by a defective system but is always due to overeating. Fat people could of course get thin by eating less but they felt utterly dreadful, tired and irritable while they were doing it. They were starving themselves, what could anyone expect?

It was true that one got fat by eating too much food, but that wasn't, MacKarness insisted, the point. The real answer lay in discovering the cause of the fat person's failure 'to use up as much as he takes in as food'. Perhaps, he speculated, it was just that the fat were greedy, or perhaps it could also be that 'although he only eats a normal amount, some defect in the way his body deals with food deflects some of what he eats to his fat stores and keeps it there instead of letting him use it up for energy'. In other words, a defective metabolism and not careless gluttony was the key. This was the beginning of the idea that obesity has a genetic cause.

The first thing to understand was that starch and sugar fattened the fat, and the real reason for excess fat was 'A DEFECTIVE CAPACITY FOR DEALING WITH CARBOHYDRATES', a failure to burn up the excess. MacKarness's use of capitals betrays his irritation with the fad diet pundits and his eagerness to put everybody straight. He credited Banting with having made this discovery a hundred years before, having dieted down by 3½ stone 'painlessly and without starvation, enjoying good food and good wine while he did it'. Banting had learned from his doctor that carbohydrates were the fat man's poison. During the twentieth century, doctors and diet experts had stuck like glue to the 'eat less/calorie-reduction' theory, a 'dogma enshrined in history and hallowed by the blessing of the high priests of modern physiological research'. But then, in 1944, came the news that the New York City Hospital had put its obese patients on diets which allowed more than twenty-four ounces of fat meat a day! They were encouraged to eat to the limit of their appetites, and some were very happy to comply – and, astonishingly, they still lost weight.

This revival of Banting's theory was put into action by Dr Blake F. Donaldson, but at the time only raised interest in America, as Britain was still in the grip of wartime rations that restricted the amounts of available fat and protein. But in 1956 the *Lancet* published the results of a study of the Banting diet carried out at London's Middlesex Hospital by Professor Alan Kerwick and Dr G. L. S. Pawan. Banting, they concluded, was right: 'The composition of the diet can alter the expenditure of calories in obese persons, increasing it when fat and proteins are given and decreasing it when carbohydrates are given.' If the proportions of fat, carbohydrate and protein were kept constant, the rate of weight loss was proportional to the calorie intake. But if the calorie intake was kept constant at 1,000 a day, the most rapid weight loss was noted with high-fat diets. If the calorie intake rose to 2,600 a day, weight loss still occurred as long as the intake was mainly in the form of fat and protein. They concluded that between 30 and 50 per cent of weight loss was derived from the total body water and the remaining 50 to 70 per cent came from body fat. Proteins, vitally important in our food but used by the body for growth and repair of tissues and muscles, don't have much effect on weight. The reduction of carbohydrate in the diet, as had long been realised, was the key to slimming down.

During the twentieth century the business of losing weight became an even greater industry than ever before. Through two world wars, and economic conditions of depression and prosperity, there were different but equally demanding pressures to be thin – all to do with, paradoxically, indulgence. Hence the rise of diet gurus such as Benjamin Gayelord Hauser and body-shapers such as Charles Atlas, both of whom favoured a regimen of discipline and strict rules. Such figures profited from the age of cinema and glamour, and from a fame industry that attracted condemnation as well as publicity for having, or being seen to have, too much during the post-war and post-depression periods. In parallel to these trends there was an advance in scientific knowledge: on the one hand, in serious research studies such as Keys's and analyses by Fishbein, MacKarness, et al., which built on the past; and on the other, the exploitation of pharmaceutical breakthroughs by profit-driven drug companies who were aware that their products brought short-term gains and long-term failures.

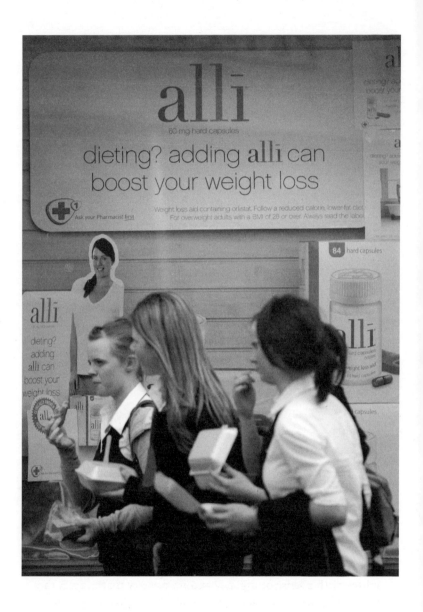

10. Today's diet industry is worth millions: we are still swallowing drugs, trying the quick fix diets, the magic bracelets and the wonder-knickers. Perhaps it's time for a re-think, to go for long-term change over short-term illusion, to step back from the dieting free-for-all and simplify our approach.

10

Modern Industrial Dieting

URING THE LAST HUNDRED YEARS the dieting busi-ness has exploded: as we have seen in the previous chapters, the market for slimming plans, drugs, foods, drinks and assorted paraphernalia has soared. Desperate means have always been a feature of the diet industry, and, while some of these have been harmless – ideas, concoctions and devices that might have hurt the pocket but not the body – some have been dangerous and occasionally fatal. Many foul and extraordinary ways to get thin have been advertised and tried – chewing gums have been laced with laxatives, cigarettes with appetite suppressants – and a lot of them were, are, just scams and tricks conjured up by doctors, charlatans and gurus. A famous face may promote the product or the feel-good marketing will feature a deliriously smiling woman in her thirties whose idea of nirvana is having the bum she had when she was seventeen. Diet books are everywhere, written with a sense of urgency and immediacy that mimics the anticipation of satisfaction. They exploit the urge for gratifica-tion and promote unattainable goals that inevitably provoke a vicious circle of self-loathing and failure.

The diet industry is all about exploitation and profit. The

slimming drugs available to us now are just the latest in a long line of imaginative, often spurious, diet preparations. Many purport to be 'natural' such as, for example, those based on the açai berry. Marketers for this diet 'phenomenon' have made scientifically unfounded claims about its efficacy, have misused celebrity names, and made assertions that açai could reverse diabetes and other chronic illnesses, and could even increase penis size as well as reduce weight. The Federal Trade Commission ('Protecting America's Consumers') has recently recovered some $25 million to settle allegations of deceptive marketing of diet products. In 2007, the FTC complained that inadequate scientific evidence had been used in TrimSpa's advertising claims that the product, and one of its ingredients, *Hoodia gordonii*, caused rapid and substantial weight loss by suppressing the appetite. The late Anna Nicole Smith had given TrimSpa's 'Ephedra-Free Formula X32' her celebrity endorsement, saying she had lost 69 pounds in just eight months. Another claim for 'Your high *speed* dream body diet pill' (my italics) ran, 'It makes losing 30, 50, even 70 pounds (or however many pounds you need to lose) painless.' The FTC Chair said, 'You won't find weight loss in a bottle of pills that claims it has the latest scientific breakthrough or miracle ingredient … paying for fad science is a good way to lose cash, not pounds.' It's a good way to lose your health and confidence, too.

In February 2009 the *Lancet* reported on a new over-the-counter obesity drug, orlistat, already approved for sale in America, and now similarly approved throughout Europe. This new diet pill sensation, which goes by the trade name Alli, 'promotes' weight loss by preventing the body from absorbing fat and is targeted at those with a BMI of 28 or higher. Making Alli as easily procurable as aspirin simply encourages the idea of a one-stop, pill-popping shortcut to getting the slim, and allegedly most desirable, body that adorns all the media. But Alli costs a lot more at your local chemist than it does on prescription: about £1.40 (US$2) per day in England against £7.40 for a monthly prescription. And, of course, the drug has only a limited effect – the average weight loss per year is just 2.5 kg. The *Lancet* points out that such easy accessibility to Alli may not be a good thing because the drug is almost guaranteed to be abused and that a lack of medical supervision could also mean that this abuse, for which read overuse, might lead to undiagnosed problems. In 2011 the FDA began investigating this 'most-studied weight loss medicine' over links to thirty-two reports of serious liver injury in patients, twenty-seven of whom were hospitalised. What we know for certain is that it has some rather unfortunate side effects that include flatulence and particularly unpleasant and colourful diarrhoea. But these minor inconveniences aren't going to stop a rush on the shops.

In early 2011 the FDA refused to approve yet another diet pill, Contrave, telling the pharmaceutical company that developed it that it must carry out long-term studies to ensure the drug will not raise the risk of heart attacks. Contrave is a combination of two existing drugs that together work to suppress food cravings: one is bupropion, an antidepressant (Wellbutrin, also sold as Zyban to help people give up smoking), the other is naltrexone, used to treat alcohol and drug addiction. The last obesity drug approved was Xenical from Roche in 1999, and that little-used drug is now the only one available for long-term use. No such drug studied so far has had a favourable side-effect profile. The FDA's latest refusal emphasises extra safety precautions because of the serious health problems of some of the older diet pills, and making it more difficult for drug companies to develop such drugs also confirms that it is lifestyle change that is really what's needed. And, anyway, Contrave, as with other weight-loss pills, has been proven to be only modestly effective, except in terms of the manufacturer's profits.

The slimming products market can be divided into five groups based on the mechanisms of action: boosting fat burning (thermogenesis), inhibiting protein breakdown, suppressing appetite and boosting feelings of fullness, blocking fat absorption, and regulating mood. Manufacturers suggest that you might, just might, if you pay out enough cash and swallow enough pills, lose just a few pounds over recommended periods, measly amounts which you could quite happily manage by not buying biscuits, and even then unlikely to be a lasting achievement. Packaging these products as 'science' is insulting and misleading, and the industry which fostered our obsession with fat is now profiting from an obesity epidemic. In Britain, prescriptions for weight-loss drugs were up by 13 per cent in 2009 to 1.45 million, an 11-fold rise in a decade. The industry is fattening itself up nicely.

Diet gurus constantly appear, too, as they have been doing for nearly two hundred years, selling their 'expertise', their regimens and special foods. The French doctor, Pierre Dukan, in a story reminiscent of Banting's over a hundred years before, created his best-selling diet after one of his overweight patients begged him for help. Dukan obliged, telling the patient to go away and eat all the non-fatty meat he liked, drink plenty of water, and come back and see him in five days. This he did, having allegedly lost ten pounds. The Dukan diet has the scientific authority required to lend credibility, and dieters are reassured that they can eat as much as they want: there is no hunger, no sacrifice to be made in terms of quantity. At first the dieter is allowed to eat as much as he or she likes, choosing from a list of seventy-two high-protein foods including lean meat, fish and a few non-fat dairy products, then vegetables are introduced (from a prescribed list of twenty-eight). The diet eschews calorie-counting and consists of four stages: two in which to lose the weight and two to maintain the loss (these are called 'attack' and 'cruise' – suitably aggressive labels). Claxton's calorie-conscious diet of 1937 also had phases, as does the Atkins diet, one of Dukan's more recent predecessors. The Atkins has four phases: Induction; Ongoing weight loss; Pre-maintenance; and Lifetime maintenance in which the dieter first gets their body used to fat and 'cures' it of cravings for 'unacceptable' foods then, gradually, carbohydrate levels are increased until a stage of weight-equilibrium is attained. According to Dukan, Atkins revolutionised diet thinking by noting that not all calories are the same, that 100 calories from sugar are very different to 100 from, say, fish, but the problem with the Atkins diet was, he argued, that it allowed you to eat as much fat as you wanted. This, Dukan says, works when you are losing weight but not when you are trying to maintain that loss.

Robert Atkins was an American cardiologist (1930–2003) who, in his early thirties, weighed 224 pounds, due largely to a junk food diet. In 1963 he read a report in the *Journal of the American Medical Association* on Alfred W. Pennington's low-starch diet and, taking his cue, he lost weight, and so did sixty-five of his patients. By 1965 Atkins was appearing on the *Tonight* show and an article on him and his diet appeared in *Vogue* in 1970 (for a while his diet was known as the 'Vogue diet'). *Dr Atkins' Diet Revolution* was published in 1972, going on to sell millions of copies and, twenty years later, *Dr Atkins' New Diet Revolution* came out and was another runaway best-seller. At the height of its popularity, in 2003 and 2004, it was estimated that one in eleven North American adults was on the diet. It is advertised as 'the no-hunger, luxurious weight loss plan that really works' and is what is known as a ketogenic diet. Ketosis is the process whereby, if you eat few carbohydrates, then there is no glucose to trigger an insulin response and the body is forced to use up its fats as a primary fuel source. Atkins argued that carbohydrates cause the body to overproduce insulin which metabolises blood glucose and makes people feel hungry. His diet restricts digestible carbohydrates as do more recent diets that come from the other angle, such as the Carb-Lover's diet. This plan allows as many carbohydrates as you like as long as they are resistant (that is, the ones that escape digestion in the small intestine). In the grand time-honoured way, the Carb-Lover's diet tells you that you can 'eat what you love and get slim for life', and that it is a 'revolutionary new science for quick and sustained weight loss'.

Atkins was another diet guru in a now long and familiar line: a fat person who discovered a diet, tried it apparently success-fully on himself, and then went on to sell it to others – and he had the added authority of being a doctor. Dukan has said that he's tried more than two hundred different diet plans (and that the only one worth a mention is Weight Watchers because it offers group support). He let his diet loose on the French public some ten years ago and his books have shifted millions of copies worldwide. He now makes much use of the internet, with about 100,000 subscribers in France alone paying about €10 a month for the privilege. Celebrity endorsement has definitely helped his business although in 2010 the French food agency, ANSES, reported that the Dukan and the Atkins diet, and others like them, could lead to muscle wastage, bone fractures and an increased risk of cancer and heart disease. Drs Lecerf and Cocaul remarked that 95 per cent of those who follow a diet plan regain weight as soon as they stop, and in some cases gain even more weight afterwards.

New diets come and go but they are always rehashed from the past, and the same goes for some of the flakier slimming products on the weight-loss market – hologram bracelets, for example, or cellulite-busting tights that melt away your fat with crystals. Scala Bio-Fir, 'new hi-tech legwear' for women, is supposed to increase blood flow and heat up the skin with a 'wonder yarn' embedded with bio-crystals, and 'could slim hips and thighs by as much as an inch'. These successors to the rubber garments and corsets of the early twentieth century are supposed to give you a 'sleeker silhouette' and it is claimed that, in tests, eight out of ten women who tried them lost fat – but they had to wear them for six hours a day for thirty days in a row. This same magic material is used in Scala Bio-Fir knickers, which broke the department store John Lewis's records with sales of 25,000 in the month after their launch. And there are new pharmaceutical developments, too, such as those involving anti-hunger smells, using particular aromas in food product development for activating areas of your brain that signal fullness; the challenge, according to the *Journal of Agricultural and Food Chemistry*, is to implement these 'concepts' into real food products. Fat-burning lip balm is another crazy innovation: the American manufacturers of Burner Balm say it will curb appetite and increase energy levels while burning fat and carbohydrates. The lip balm contains green tea and *Hoodia* extract, thought to be appetite suppressants, but the National Obesity Forum has condemned the product as a damaging gimmick aimed at young girls.

What about bribery as an incentive to lose the extra weight? An NHS primary care trust in Kent offered cash rewards of up to £425 on a year-long 'Pounds for Pounds' trial in 2009. It reported that of the 402 volunteers who went on the scheme more than a hundred of them lost nearly 2 stone each in a year. But the high drop-out rate meant that the true impact of a cash reward was unclear. The scheme was run by a private company, Weight Wins, which also offers a payout of thousands of pounds to private customers who lose a certain amount of weight over a certain amount of time and keep it off for a prescribed period, too. Customers pay a joining fee for the scheme with a monthly subscription thereafter and, of course, if you don't succeed you're out of pocket (again). Cash isn't everyone's motivational cup of tea so you could go to the Fat Whisperer of West Hollywood, a weight-loss guru who talks to her client's fat cells, encouraging them to leave the body. 'I command you to get out!' she is reported to order the unwanted cells, like a latterday cleansing of the Temple. To back up her technique of fat persuasion she also uses her own low-calorie diet, detoxifying masks, teas and wraps, heated inflatable suits and an ultrasound machine: all the rigmarole one might expect, and up to 70 per cent of her business is, apparently, celebrity-based.

To the individual, fat is a personal problem rather than a public one, but it has also figured powerfully as a national concern, even before the present obsession with an obesity crisis. In times of economic depression and war, fat people have been singled out as traitors, especially during the First and Second World Wars, but it goes back much further. Government public health interventions and broad, community-based plans have encouraged people to lose weight as a civic duty – a notion that originates in classical antiquity. As recently as January 2011, the *Boston Globe* argued that prevention of obesity by a sophisticated and aggressive federal approach is the only viable answer to the obesity epidemic. In Britain, millions of pounds were spent on the Change4Life Campaign, a society-wide movement to prevent people getting fat in the first place. A French scheme has everyone from shop owners, teachers, doctors, pharmacists, restaurant owners, sports associations, the media, scientists and local government joining in, in an effort to encourage children to eat better and run around more. Two Swedish studies have suggested that cognitive therapy – which teaches people the mental and emotional skills they need to make and sustain change – helps people to regulate their emotions and control their eating habits.

The dieting habits that daughters acquire from their mothers may not just be something they have learned. The genetic hypothesis, one of the latest reassessments of the obesity problem, suggests that a strong hereditary predisposition to fat can go back several decades. People who are morbidly obese (those with a BMI of at least 40) are said to lack a tiny stretch of DNA that contains around thirty genes, according to the investigation released in 2010 by *Nature* magazine. No one is yet clear, though, what it is that the missing genes actually do, and other genetic gaps or variations involved in chronic obesity may yet be uncovered. The genes that are linked to weight gain, and there could be hundreds, each contributing a very small amount to variation in weight, have not been shown so far to have much effect on fat accumulation, just a kilo (two pounds) or less. The individual's response to environment, to junk food, say, or exercise is genetically based, too. The conclusion is that across all ages around 70 per cent of the variability of adiposity and fat distribution within the population is attributable to heritable genetic differences, and around 30 per cent to environmental differences. Despite these evolutionary and biological influences, most scientists in the field agree that the increasing obesity rates seen in many countries during the late twentieth century do not result from internal changes, but from people's environmental changes, where they choose what and how much they eat and move. The food industry, some scientists argue, has engineered its products to appeal to our biological cravings for substances that increase our risk for major chronic diseases – calorie-dense, nutrient-poor food is more and more available, less expensive, and more appealingly packaged, worldwide. Like the tobacco and alcohol industries, most food and drink companies lay the emphasis on individual responsibility when it comes to our sweet, salty and fatty pleasures, so that the health-related costs of their products can be dumped straight back on to the consumers and the tax-payers.

Social and cultural influences have led many dieters to pick a target weight outside their 'set point' weight range, one which they are unlikely to maintain and never without a good deal of misery. In the mid-1990s, Jeffrey M. Friedman, a molecular geneticist at Rockefeller University, discovered the appetite-regulating hormone leptin and argued that this can cause overweight people to have different 'set points' of weight at different times in their lives. Many scientists believe that people are genetically programmed to maintain their weight within a set-point range that varies from person to person regardless of other similarities like height. This suggests the best explanation for the body's resistance to losing weight. Set-point theory says that being overweight and underweight should be understood in terms of being above or below the individual's set point. A very thin woman, they say, may appear underweight but this could be appropriate for her body, being at or above her set point. This argument has its supporters and its detractors, but it is known that overweight people 'defend their fat stores as rigorously as those of normal weight'. That is not to say that an individual's set point won't be influenced by age, diet and exercise habits or whether or not they smoke and drink – if you do a lot of exercise your set point could become lower, but if you eat too much fat and sugar it could rise. And, crucially, dieting seems to promote a higher set point.

The food choices we make from what's on offer to us, the psychology of our decision-making processes, directly impacts on the physiological effects of our diet. Pharmacologists, physiologists, geneticists, economists, sociologists and psychologists are all busy looking into our innate preferences and learned food aversions. People who like the taste of a doughnut (good) but worry about their weight (bad), experience these conflicting responses simultaneously and those with high ambivalence are more easily persuaded to give in to food temptation. We say that the health benefits of certain foods are important to us but research suggests that manufacturers, having improved the taste of low-fat alternatives, are more successful when they appeal directly to our interest in weight loss.

One way to change behaviour and choice is just to imagine your way through it. Seriously: just thinking about eating something instead of actually consuming it could help change your diet and habits. A study of more than three hundred volunteers, published in *Science*, maintains that going through the mental motions of eating, say, a bar of chocolate, will help you re-set the way you eat. And the study suggests the technique could help, too, with cravings for other substances such as tobacco and alcohol. Trying to stop yourself thinking about food when you are on a diet is almost impossible as well as miserable, but repeatedly allowing yourself to imagine the actual eating, taste and swallowing, rather than just suppressing the thought of it or trying to distract yourself, apparently leads to less of the actual food being consumed, up to 50 per cent less, according to the findings. The study looked at the neurological process of 'habituation', and discovered that it is not just governed by the sensory inputs of sight, smell, sound and touch, but also by how the consumption experience is mentally represented. Merely imagining an experience seems to be a substitute for the actual experience. Different foods arouse both emotional and cognitive responses, and both our heart and our head are involved in choosing what and how much we eat – a change of mood may be a direct result of what we eat, and sometimes we even consciously seek it out. We've all surely recognised that sweet and fatty tastes have influenced our moods, good and bad, and that we have specifically chosen to eat chocolate, for example, to do just that.

Eating activates areas in the brain in a similar way to drugs such as opiates. It is thought that dopamine, a neurotransmitter that among other actions causes intense pleasure, is behind the motivational aspects of wanting, and so of eating. Sensitivity to reward has been found to be lower in obese people than in slightly overweight people, suggesting that many chronically overeat in order to stimulate the release of more dopamine. This could also help with the misery of the social stigma of eating if you are very fat, as dopamine alleviates stress and depression. It may also be relevant that eating disorders, such as binge eating, are associated with a greater risk of drug abuse. It is possible that people overeat because they are confusing emotional arousal with hunger and, or, hoping to comfort or distract themselves from emotional distress with food. Although this may sound a little obvious, it has only been the subject of serious research for the last thirty years or so. A study in 1983 analysing mood ratings found that overweight women ate more snacks during bad than good moods. In 1998, a trial with nurses and teachers who completed diet diaries found that they upped their high-fat intake when their stress levels were at their highest. And in 2002 another study found that reward-related eating was linked to an enhanced release of dopamine – association by repetition. From these results, however, comes an argument for the development of drugs aimed at blocking the pleasant dopamine effects of particular foods. Effectively, they will remove the pleasure one gets from eating (the opposite of the earlier use of Benzedrine). It is the giving of drugs to stop the effect of drugs.

This is part of the medicalisation of our society, where all kinds of behaviours and conditions previously accepted as human variations are now regarded as a profitable open market for pharmaceutical companies. So, for example, extremely shy people might be prescribed drugs for party-going, and fat people to make them thin because, obviously, the truly ideal person is confident and THIN. This idea isn't new either. Doctors such as Leonid Kotkin, for instance, who wrote *Eat, Think and Be Slender* in 1954, opined that therapists and doctors could get 'a good deal of pleasure watching the real self emerge from the fatty shell'. The radical psychiatrist Thomas Szasz argued in 1973 that his profession was created to study and control people who didn't fit the medical 'norms' of social behaviour. In the past, according to Szasz, it targeted homosexuals, Jews, drug addicts and the insane, and now it was beginning to include the over-weight and to impose diets and regimens as a moral order as well as, or rather than, any sort of scientific answer. A new specialisa-tion, bariatrics (from the Greek *baros* – weight), was created in the mid-1960s to describe those who were the 'wrong' weight and, as Szasz noted, within a short space of time, by 1972, the newly created American Society of Bariatric Physicians had 450 members. Another psychiatrist, Albert J. Stunkard, also writing in 1973, claimed that, 'During the past twenty-five years inter-est in weight reduction in our country has grown from a mild concern to an overriding preoccupation. At present, interest in obesity almost assumes the dimensions of a national neurosis.'

This looks like a neurosis that isn't going to go away in a hurry. Even just thinking you might be a bit overweight can cause an inordinate amount of worry for some people, and it has been estimated that at least one in every two women who are not deemed to be overweight has been on a diet. Whether a dieter reaches and maintains his or her goal is often explained in terms of personality type or other psychological constructs. Most people, even professionals, believe that the overweight can diet successfully if only they would try hard enough, but the difference between success and failure is not to be explained by one single phenomenon. We know that there are physiological changes that occur when we eat less than we need, and there is increasing evidence that dieters get locked into a circular struggle with their own system as it attempts to deal with the starvation process. The gradually decreasing weight loss that is experienced after the first stage of dieting makes it more and more difficult to keep going.

The actual effect of any particular diet is minuscule but the effect of individual behaviour is enormous, according to a major study on 800 overweight American adults reported in *The New*

England Journal of Medicine in 2009. Some people in the study lost fifty pounds while others gained five, so the important question, according to Dr F. M. Sacks at the Harvard School of Public Health, is what biological, psychological or social factors influence whether a person can stick to any diet? In the future, said Sacks, researchers should focus less on the actual diet and more on finding out what is the main reason for success. Addressing your psyche, individually and collectively, is the main thing. Diets only tackle symptoms and can make you feel worse because you will probably fail … unless you take a good long look at how your mind is working.

Motivation and commitment to lose weight are only part of the question. According to psychologists at the University of Toronto, if a dieter's resolve is undermined by a slip which temporarily releases them from their vows of abstinence then, instead of doing penance for the calorific sin, they will persist in 'bad' indulgence. To think, as many do, that 'one may as well be hung for a sheep as a lamb' is a seductive thought process, a trap which all dieters can fall into. If you've 'failed' and had one piece of cake, why not have the whole thing, ditch the diet for the day and start again tomorrow? And, in anticipation of self-inflicted deprivation, dieters indulging on 'the night before' can really go to town. By denying themselves food, it becomes much more important to them than it was before. Dieters, as we have seen, are more likely than non-dieters to turn to food when anxious or depressed. They don't eat interminably once their rules are broken but they eat far more than non-dieters do. And, apparently, a vital element influencing a dieter's success is 'emotional readiness', meaning that in order for a diet to be successful one has to go into training for it, much as you might for a marathon run. Preparation and planning are all.

When you begin a diet you make a conscious decision to lose weight and you override your automatic internal regulators. So if you break your diet, either temporarily or for good, you run the risk of rebound binge eating. And as you diet, your body will adjust itself to survive on less energy and your metabolic rate (the rate at which we use up energy) goes down. The more weight is lost the less food is needed, which can also make you lethargic and slow down your metabolic rate. If you lose weight too quickly you could be losing lean tissue or muscle as well as fat and, as your metabolic rate is determined by the amount of lean tissue you have, it could reduce your metabolic rate even further. So the general advice is that it's best to plan carefully and lose weight slowly: a life-long commitment is called for instead of going from one diet to another in a repetitive fashion. This type of repetitive dieting risks one's health, possibly more so than just staying slightly overweight. It has been linked to cardiovascular disease, stroke, diabetes – all on the rise in the Western world – though scientists don't yet fully understand how.

The *New England Journal of Medicine* carried a study on men and women whose weight fluctuated a great deal over a period of many years and found that they had a significantly higher risk of death, particularly from heart disease, than those with a relatively stable weight, even if that was quite high. In the UK there are up 30,000 premature and avoidable deaths through obesity each year – and the NHS spends around £1 billion a year on treating it, with a further £2.3 billion of indirect costs. More than half the people in Europe are overweight or obese and Britons are the fattest of the lot – obesity in the UK has trebled during the last twenty-five years, meaning that almost one in four adults and an estimated one in five children are overweight. In America, the figures are two-thirds of adults and one-third of children. The *Journal of the American Medical Association* says that if this continues, as looks likely, then obesity will account for more than $860 billion – over 16 per cent of healthcare expenditure in the United States – by 2030. Medical costs over an American lifetime for someone who is seventy pounds or more overweight are said to be up to $30,000. There are warnings, too, that obesity could overtake alcohol as the main cause of liver cirrhosis, and that most people are just not aware that this disease is associated with excess weight.

Dieting changes the way we feel about our body, encouraging overly critical evaluations of body shape and size. Several studies, such as Ancel Keys's into cholesterol, have shown how dieting changes the relationship with food, producing powerful urges to eat, excessive preoccupation with, and feelings of being out of control around, food, all leading to a vulnerability to temptation. Dieters can get locked into this distorted relationship, get out of touch with their normal appetite, and may only be able to maintain some semblance of control within the guidelines of a diet plan. And they score higher than non-dieters on measures of emotional agitation and are more likely to show impaired mental performance – the stress of restricting your food is continual and damaging. According to psychologists, people, mainly women and girls, who suffer such psychological distress from dieting patterns need help to give them up and to re-evaluate the attitudes that have created their body-insecurity. India Knight and Neris Thomas, authors of *Idiot-Proof Diet* (2007), recognise this from personal experience and they run an online forum that addresses these issues. They acknowledge self-loathing, the sense of shame, the insecurity, the guilt, the issues around sex, the despair, the ugly, violent language women use about their own bodies, and the timid longing: 'Can I really do it? Will it really work?' To remedy all of the above by losing weight can be overwhelmingly affecting and addresses something that has blighted every aspect of their lives, sometimes for decades, sometimes from childhood. In this approach, bullying is out and support is in, along with the idea that it is not unfeminist, unintelligent or vain to regain control of your life. There is no single, right way of looking at ourselves and at the space we occupy in the minds of others. It's all, as they say, in the eye of the beholder, and the way that beholder sees changes, too, in place and time. What we think of as facts are, like body shapes, mutable.

The group support approach to slimming is not new but it is very successful. In America it has been big business and attracted extraordinary numbers. In 1952 the US Public Health Service convened a national conference on the Group Approach to Weight Control and, around the same time, Esther Manz adopted the Alcoholics Anonymous method, a strategy that works for many thousands, and began the first national diet group, TOPS – Take Off Pounds Sensibly – which had 30,000 members by 1958 and had doubled that by 1963. Local groups sprang up calling themselves by such names as Invisi-Belles, Inches Anonymous, Shrinking Violets, Thick 'N Tired, WADS (We Are Dieting Seriously), SIRENS (Slenderness Is Right Endeavors Never Stop). Overeaters Anonymous began in 1960, Weight Watchers in 1963, Diet Workshop, Inc. in 1965. Two studies from the Medical Research Council, led by Susan Jebb, one of Britain's leading nutrition scientists, say that Weight Watchers – which once referred to itself as a 'behaviour-modification' programme – can really work, and is a cheap and effective way for the NHS to tackle Britain's serious obesity problem. Other recent studies in Europe and America have concurred. In a trial of some 800 people using different diets, fewer people dropped out among those who joined Weight Watchers, though the drop-out rate was high. Those who completed a year of Weight Watchers lost around 7 kg each, nearly twice as much as those being managed by their doctor. It is also the case that 90 per cent of the dieters were women, leading to suggestions that the group approach just doesn't appeal to men. But in the first decades of Alcoholics Anonymous most of the alcoholics who came to the meetings were men (female alcoholics were up against a greater stigmatisation) and it is possible that many men simply feel that dieting is 'unmanly'. We only have to look at the rise in interest in male grooming, however, to see that this is very likely to change. The key thing about the group approach is support.

In a *Scientific American* article of February 2011, David H. Freedman discussed how behavioural analysts looking at diets had long recognised some basic conditions which gave a greater chance of losing weight and keeping it off. His four steps to losing weight are:

1. Determine your baseline measurements – how much do you weigh? What rituals and routines contribute to your overeating or under-exercising?
2. Make small changes first – use stairs instead of lifts, look at the food on the table to see what is on offer before filling your plate.
3. Record your body weight, count the calories, log your progress and seek objective feedback.
4. Use support groups, real or virtual, share successes and setbacks and plan strategies.

If dieters measure and record calories, exercise and weight, if they make modest and gradual changes rather than severe ones, if they make wise choices over the foods they eat and have a balanced diet, low on fats and sugar, high on vegetables, fruit and wholegrains and don't avoid major food groups, if they set themselves clear and modest goals, look to lifelong habits rather than fad diets, and if they join dieting groups which offer encouragement, support and praise, then their efforts are much more likely to succeed. It has to become second nature, you have to re-habituate yourself into a lifelong change of diet and behaviour but, according to a recent report in the *New England Journal of Medicine*, it doesn't usually need that great a change: 'A handful of the right lifestyle changes will go a long way.'

A study of diets over the centuries reveals one trend in particular: that of the once very fat person (or, better still, a slimmed-down doctor whose overweight patients implore him or her for help) who devises a diet which is startlingly successful and goes on to market it to the rest of the world with books, plans, foods and colourful endorsements. This trend we can trace through Cornaro, Banting, Atkins and Dukan, ad infinitum. They commonly propose a structured diet with specific stages one must follow, first to lose the weight and then to maintain the loss by making careful food choices, being active and embracing moderation. Divested of the personalities, the magical thinking and the sometimes inordinate costs, this long-term, balanced and low-carbohydrate approach – in short, taking care of the whole – is the way to go. If the dieter has support as well, they are much more likely to succeed. It's a slow process, made more difficult by our habituation to instant gratification and a luxurious variety of foods. Psychologists say that you need to use 'double think' – to be optimistic about achieving your goal but also realistic about some of the barriers that stand in your way. What we need is a different emphasis, and one that moves firmly away from ingrained notions of failure and weakness. We can't, and shouldn't, remove the story of diets from the story of health, but we can do something about the weight of judgement and the smear of sin and temptation. The truth is that today's quick-fix fad dieting is never going to work. We must think again, and radically, about gratification. What we need to do is return to the ancient Greek philosophy of *diaita*, bring it up to date for twenty-first-century living, and remember Cornaro's sixteenth-century 'first rule': that we must regain control and cease to be slaves to passions which turn out to be no more than delusions.

Bibliography

Primary Texts

Anon., A Minister of the Interior, *Memoirs of a Stomach, Written By Himself, That All Who Eat May Read* ... (W. E. Painter, 1853)

Anon., A Physician, *Advice on Diet and Regime* (London, 1820)

Anon., D— S— , *Advice to Stout People: Showing How I Reduced from 20 Stone to 13 Stone with Full Particulars As to Diet, Treatment, Etc.* (George Routledge & Sons, 1883)

Armstrong, John, *The Art of Preserving Health: A Poem* (A. Millar, 1747)

Banting, William, *Letters on Corpulence, Addressed to the Public* (London, 1863)

Beard, George, *Eating and Drinking* (New York, 1871)

Bell, Robert, *The Secret of Long Life* (David Bryce & Son, 1894)

Blake, Edward, *Constipation and Some Associated Disorders* (G. P. Putnam & Sons, 1900)

Boorde, Andrew, *A Breviary of Health* (W. Powell, c.1552)

Bradshaw, Watson, *On Corpulence* (London, 1864)

Brillat-Savarin, Jean Anthelme, *The Handbook of Dining or Corpulency and Leanness Scientifically Considered* (J. C. Nimmo & Bain, 1884)

Brillat-Savarin, Jean Anthelme, *The Physiology of Taste or Meditations on Transcendental Gastronomy* (Penguin Classic, 2004; first published, 1825)

Chesser, Eustace, *Slimming for the Million: The New Treatment of Obesity: A Practical Guide for Patient and Physician* (London, 1939)

Cheyne, George, *An Essay on Regimen* (London, 1742)

Claxton, E. E., with recipes by Lucy Burdekin, *Weight Reduction: Diet and Dishes* (W. Heinemann Ltd, 1937)

Cogan, Thomas, *The Haven of Health ... amplified upon five words of Hippocrates* (London, 1584)

Cornaro, Luigi, *Sure and Certain Methods of Attaining a Long and Healthful Life* (Daniel Midwinter, 1722)

Cornaro, Luigi, *The Art of Living Long: A New and Improved English Version of the Treatise of the Celebrated Venetian Centenarian Louis Cornaro with Essays by Joseph Addison, Lord Bacon, and Sir William Temple* (W. F. Butler, 1903)

Craston, George Henry, *Pretty Faces and How They Are Made, Without Paint, Rouges, Cosmetics, or Any Artificial Means: How Everybody Can Be Pretty* (T. Ashworth, 1896)

Davies, Nathaniel Edward, *Food for the Fat: A Treatise on Corpulency with Dietary for its Cure* (Chatto, 1891)

Dutton, Thomas, *Indigestion: Gout, Corpulency and Constipation* (Henry Kimpton, 1892)

Elyot, Thomas, *The Castel of Helth Gathered and Made ... out of the Chiefe Authors of Physycke ... that he be not deceyued* (London, 1534)

Fishbein, Morris, *Your Diet and Your Health* (McGraw-Hill, 1937)

Fishbein, Morris (ed.), *Your Weight and How to Control It: A Scientific Guide by Medical Specialists and Dieticians Including the Principles of Nutrition, with Diets and Menus for Reducing and Gaining* (Doubleday Doran & Co., 1929)

Fitch, William Edward, *Dietotherapy* (D. Appleton & Co., 1918)

Frumusan, Jean, *The Cure of Obesity* translated from the French (J. Bale, Sons & Danielsson Ltd., 1924)

Hauser, Bengamin Gayelord, *Eat and Grow Beautiful* (Faber & Faber, 1939)

Hauser, Bengamin Gayelord, *Look Younger, Live Longer* (London, Faber and Faber, 1951)

Hornibrook, Frederick, *The Culture of the Abdomen: The Cure of Obesity and Constipation* (London, 1933)

Huack, Hazel, M., *How to Control Your Weight* (New York, 1942)

Hunt Peters, Lulu, *Dieting and Health: With Key to the Calories* (Cornell University Library, 2009; first published 1918)

Kellogg, John Harvey, *Rational Hydrotherapy* (London, 1900)

Keys, Ancel, *The Biology of Human Starvation* (University of Minnesota Press, 1950)

Leyel, C. F., *Diet and Commonsense* (Chatto & Windus, 1936)

Lieb, Clarence, *Eat, Drink, and Be Slender: What Every Overweight Person Should Know and Do* (New York, 1929)

MacKarness, Richard, *Eat Fat and Grow Slim* (Harvill, 1958)

Markham, Gervase, *Hunger's Prevention* (A. Mathewes, 1621)

Moffett, Thomas, *Health's Improvement* (London, 1655)

Moore, A. W., *Corpulency; I.e. Fat, or, Embonpoint, in Excess: Letters to the Medical Times and Gazette … Explaining Briefly his Newly-Discovered DIET SYSTEM, to Reduce the Weight and Benefit the Health* (J. Sheppard, 1856)

Roskruge, A. M. S., *The Cloven Hoof: An Epic for Epicures, and a Philosophical Text Book Containing the Secret of Long Life* (The Ideal Publishing Union, 1895)

Rout, Ettie, *Sex and Exercise: A Study of the Sex Function in Women and its Relation to Exercise* (London, 1925)

Shelley, Percy Bysshe, *Oedipus Tyrannus, or, Swellfoot the Tyrant* (London, 1820)

Simmonds, Rose M., *Handbook of Diets* (W. Heinemann Ltd, 1931)

Stanford Read, C., *Fads and Feeding* (Methuen & Co., 1908)

Trotter, Thomas, *A View of the Nervous Temperament* (London, 1807)

Turner, Dorothea, *Handbook of Diet Therapy* for the American Dietetic Association (University of Chicago Press, 1946)

Vaughan, William, *Directions for Health, Naturall and Artificial, Derived From the Best Phisitians, as well Moderne as Antient* (London, John Beale, 1626)

Wadd, William, *Cursory Remarks on Corpulence or Obesity Considered as a Disease* (London, 1810)

Wadd, William, S., *The Conquest of Constipation* (London, 1923)

Walsh, William, *The Conquest of Constipation* (London, 1923)

Webb-Johnson, Cecil, *Why Be Fat?* (London, Mills & Boon, 1923)

Weir Mitchell, Silas, *Fat and Blood: and How to Make them* (Philadelphia, 1877)

Williams, Leonard, *Obesity* (London, New York, Humphrey Milford Oxford University Press, 1926)

Weir Mitchell, Silas, *Fat and Blood: and How to Make them* (Philadelphia, 1887)

Secondary Texts

Blackman, Lisa, *The Body: The Key Concepts* (Berg, 2008)

Boehrer, Bruce Thomas, *The Fury of Men's Gullets: Ben Jonson and the Digestive Canal* (University of Pennsylvania Press, 1997)

Brumberg, Joan Jacobs, *Fasting Girls: The Emergence of Anorexia Nervosa as a Modern Disease* (Harvard University Press, 1988)

Douglas, Mary, *Implicit Meanings: Selected Essays in Social Anthropology (Collected Works vol. v)* (Routledge, 1999)

Foucault, Michel, edited by Gordon, Colin, *Power/Knowledge: Selected Interviews and Other Writings 1972–1977* (Pantheon Books, c.1980)

Freedman, Paul (ed.), *Food: The History of Taste* (Thames & Hudson, 2007)

Garnsey, Peter, *Food, Health, and Culture in Classical Antiquity* (Cambridge Department of Classics Working Papers, No. 1, 1989)

Garrison, Daniel H. (ed.), *A Cultural History of the Human Body in Antiquity* (Berg, 2010)

Grant, Mark, *Galen on Food and Diet* (Routledge, 2000)

Grogan, Sarah, *Body Image: Understanding Body Dissatisfaction in Men, Women and Children* (Routledge, 2008)

Guerrini, Anita, *Obesity and Depression in the Enlightenment: The Life and Times of George Cheyne* (University of Oklahoma Press, 2000)

Hamann, Brigitte, trans. Ruth Hein, *The Reluctant Empress* (Knopf, 1986)

Haslam, D. and F., *Fat, Gluttony and Sloth: Obesity in Literature, Art and Medicine* (Liverpool University Press, 2009)

Kalof, Linda (ed.), *A Cultural History of the Human Body in the Medieval Age* (Berg, 2010)

Kalof, Linda, and Bynum, William (eds.), *A Cultural History of the Human Body in the Renaissance* (Berg, 2010)

Morton, Timothy, *Shelley and the Revolution in Taste: The Body and the Natural World* (Cambridge University Press, 1994)

Morton, Timothy (ed.), *Cultures of Taste/Theories of Appetite: Eating Romanticism* (Palgrave Macmillan, 2004)

Mullett, Charles F., edited and with an introduction by, *The Letters of Dr. George Cheyne to the Countess of Huntingdon* (Huntingdon Library, 1940)

Nasser, M., Baistow, K., and Treasure, J. (eds.), *The Female Body in Mind. The Interface between the Female Body and Mental Health* (Routledge, 2007)

Oddy, Derek J., Atkins, Peter J., and Amilien, Virginie, *The Rise of Obesity in Europe: A Twentieth Century Food History* (Ashgate, 2009)

Orbach, Susie, *Fat is a Feminist Issue: The Anti-diet Guide to Permanent Weight Loss* (Paddington Press, 1978)

Porter, Roy, *Mind-Forg'd Manacles: A History of Madness in England from the Restoration to the Regency* (Penguin, 1990)

Precope, John, *Hippocrates on Diet and Hygiene* (Zeno, 1952)

Reeves, Carole (ed.), *A Cultural History of the Human Body in the Enlightenment* (Berg, 2010)

Schwartz, Hillel, *Never Satisfied: A Cultural History of Diets, Fantasies and Fat* (Macmillan, 1986)

Shepherd, Richard, and Raats, Monique (eds.), *The Psychology of Food Choice* (CABI, 2006)

Steele, Valerie, *The Corset: A Cultural History* (Yale University Press, 2001)

Thirsk, Joan, *Food in Early Modern England: Phases, Fads, Fashions 1500–1760* (Continuum, 2009)

Trelawny, Edward John (ed. David Wright), *Records of Shelley, Byron, and the Author* (Penguin, 1973)

Journals and newspapers
The Boston Globe; Guardian; Independent; Lancet; The New York Times; Observer; Punch; Sunday Times; The Times,

Illustration Credits

1. Beth Ditto © Getty Images.
2. Hohle Fels Venus © Hilde Jensen, University of Tübingen.
3. Barbara Gammage, Countess of Leicester, wife of Robert Sidney, Earl of Leicester, and her Children, Marcus Gheeraerts (1596).
4. James Gillray, *A Voluptuary Under the Horrors of Digestion* (1792).
5. Daniel Lambert (1770–1809) © Wellcome Library, London.
6. Figuroids advert, *Windsor Magazine* (1908) © Wellcome Library, London.
7. The American Tobacco Company's Lucky Strike cigarette adverts © Advertising Archives.
8. Mother and daughter in weighing scales advert © Advertising Archives.
9. Jane Russell © Hulton Archive/Getty Images.
10. Alli weightloss pills © Jeff J Mitchell/Getty Images.

Acknowledgments

Thank you to Lizzie Speller, Fiona Green, Marcia Schofield, Ian Patterson, Sophia Wickham, Sarah Caro, Lisa Owens and Patrick Walsh.

Index